Pilgrims

Born in New Zealand, Paul McDermott now lives in London, where he has a private psychotherapy practice, and pursues his interests in Oriental philosophy and Wushu.

Pilgrims

The extraordinary story of an unlikely friendship

Paul McDermott

RIDER

LONDON · SYDNEY · AUCKLAND · JOHANNESBURG

1 3 5 7 9 10 8 6 4 2

First published in 2005 by Rider.

This paperback edition first published in 2006 by Rider,
an imprint of Ebury Press, Random House,
20 Vauxhall Bridge Road, London SW1V 2SA

Random House Australia (Pty) Limited
20 Alfred Street, Milsons Point, Sydney,
New South Wales 2061, Australia

Random House New Zealand Limited
18 Poland Road, Glenfield,
Auckland 10, New Zealand

Random House South Africa (Pty) Limited
Isle of Houghton, Corner of Boundary Road & Carse O'Gowrie
Houghton 2198, South Africa

The Random House Group Limited Reg. No. 954009

Papers used by Rider are natural, recyclable products
made from wood grown in sustainable forests.

Typeset by Palimpsest Book Production Limited,
Polmont, Stirlingshire

Printed and bound in Great Britain by
Cox & Wyman Ltd, Reading, Berks

A CIP catalogue record for this book
is available from the British Library

ISBN 1846040167 (until Jan 2007)
ISBN 9781846040160 (from Jan 2007)

In order to protect the privacy of some of the individuals mentioned
in this book, certain names have been changed.

THIS BOOK IS DEDICATED TO

EVELYN 'VAL' HALL

Behold, you showed me a mystery;
We shall all sleep,
But we shall not all be changed.

&

LAUREN ZOE and LOUIS GEORGE

Child! Do throw this book about;
Do not refrain from the holy pleasure
Of cutting all but pictures out.

CONTENTS

*You listened, not like a priest who listens for sin,
but like a sinner, who listens for his own redemption.*

Anne Michaels, *Fugitive Pieces*

Val Hall was one of my teachers. I never learn much from people telling me things. But, if I've experienced what I need to learn, then it goes in. If it was a painful lesson it tends to stick. I learned a lot from Val Hall.

I also learn from dreams. How I came to be with Val was born from three dreams. The first was the earliest dream I can remember clearly. I was around seven years of age, ill and fitfully asleep on the floor beside my mother's bed. I dreamed vividly of countless people who walked to and from the moon on my body. This was happening while I was being paraded in a white Cadillac convertible, along streets lined with thousands of cheering people.

I was being raised a Catholic, and my dream had a similar theme to the first dream in the Bible, Jacob's ladder: angels climbing to and from the heavens. I was, in this way, a bridge.

In some cultures the moon is the first stopping off place for the recently deceased. Not 'ceased', but 'de-ceased', which literally means *one who reverses having gone away*. The dream was hopeful and joyous. It had a religious intensity and an innocence that exemplified the experience I was to have with Val. I would not trade a single despairing moment spent in her company for a happy one without her.

The second dream told me I should write about Val, and provided the title of this book. It was dreamed by a colleague of mine, Debbie Charles, and begins:

> I am sitting with Paul McDermott and he hands me a book called *The Story of my Life*. It is a beautiful, hardcover book, square and perfectly bound. I went to give it back to him, and he said, 'No, it's for you,' and I was really moved by this. I went to show A. and he said, 'This is his second book. His first was a paperback called *Pilgrims*.'

On hearing this title, *Pilgrims*, I had a further glimpse into my experiences with Val. These further glimpses continue more than ten years after I met her.

So I wrote. I didn't know if I could write, but my relationship to dreams is such that I felt compelled to do it. And when I began writing, I dreamed the third dream, that of a woman approaching me with a message. I was about to give a lecture on death and dying, and the woman came right up to me and said in a warm reassuring voice, 'Just tell them what happened.' This I have attempted to do.

What follows is the true story of an extraordinary ordinary woman. Although it is *her* story, in the end it will also be yours, no matter how you, the central protagonist, may try to direct it. Death is the fundamental mystery of our lives; it is the unique individual experience; it is also the given, the inevitable fatal rite of passage and outcome of all that has gone before. And I approach this Great Mystery not as an expert, but in accord with Albert Einstein who, when asked his profession on first entering the United States, declared himself a student. It is in this vein that I have written, and it is the only honest way I can live.

INTRODUCTION

Val wrote the following shortly before she died:

Information about me (Evelyn Hall)

I was born in the King's Road, Chelsea, London SW3, illegitimately, on 1 March 1919, Evelyn Turner, and went to the National Children's Home, London. Was adopted by Mrs June and Mr Henry Clay, although not until I was fourteen years of age. I appeared before a judge, who suggested as I had only one name, I might like to choose another Christian name and he offered my natural mother's names (Amelia Grace), but I didn't like them and asked to be called Valerie (after a character in a story I was reading).

I passed the primary school scholarship when I was eleven years of age and the National School Certificate with credits in some subjects. I left school (Aldershot County High School) when I was sixteen years of age and applied to the Aldershot Post Office for a post in 1935. I used to go to a great many dances at the YMCA and the army barracks, where I met my husband to be when I was seventeen. His name was Tommy Charles Hall and he lived at 30 Gordon Road, Aldershot. Tom had a mother (Hilda Parker) and a grandmother (Sarah Blanche Backaller) who worked at Gale and Polden, and an aunt Mrs Amelia Laura Herd. Tom's grandmother was called 'Dear' by everyone and everyone loved her. I was the relief clerk for the South of England and at Bovington camp when war broke out in 1939. Tommy was in the REME (Royal Electrical and Mechanical Engineers) within a few days. He joined up in Portsmouth.

I was a teleprinter operator during the war, working mainly at night. (I had been trained at CTO where I became quite proficient).

We became engaged at Christmas 1939. Our marriage was not until 1942 – on April Fool's Day at the Red Church, at 10 a.m. By this time Tom was a sergeant.

Tom became an armourer and took an interest in armoury. Not until after his death did I discover that he had been a 'bit of a hero'. He had some troops out on the ranges when a phiat gun exploded and he threw himself on top of another soldier and, who knows, may have saved the soldier's sight. Tom was one of the 6th Airborne Paratroopers and was very, very proud of his red beret, and so was I.

At the Battle of the Bulge, he was sent to Germany and went through to Brussels. He was demobbed in January 1946. It wasn't until 1952 that I became pregnant. My daughter was born in Farnham Hospital between 5.15 a.m. and 5.30 a.m. It was not a very easy confinement, as the doctors said I had piles as big as the baby's head and have suffered from them ever since.

My daughter was a lovely blonde child but quite shy in lots of ways. She went to the same school as I had done (The Church of England School, better known as the 'National'), and then gained a scholarship to the County High School. Her name is Christine Anne, and she nearly died when she was five weeks old. I couldn't stop her screaming and eventually sent for the doctor who sent her back to Farnham Hospital where she was operated on by Dr Roare for a suspected intussusception, but apparently it straightened itself out under anaesthetic. He said that she had a thickened pyloric valve, but he decided not to cut it to save trouble when she was older. (Result – a very bad stomach scar, made by the sister who stitched her up.)

Christine worked in Barclays Bank in Guildford before leaving home and going to live in Richmond, Surrey, but she wanted to work in computers and so decided to emigrate to the USA. I don't know anything about her life out there as she is not a good correspondent. I am sorry Christine can't talk about my terminal illness (called multiple myeloma, which is a type of cancer of the blood). If only Christine could come home (to England) just for a few days to sit and talk face to face – it is my one last wish. I just hoped to get a little support from her at the time I most need it.

I think the worst contact she ever made was with her

psychoanalyst instead of a psychotherapist. I hope she
has the chance to speak to my hospice home support
visitor. I don't know how I would have managed
without relying on my many friends.

. . . One last message to my daughter. Please forgive
me for all the wrongs that I have caused you, real and
imaginary, and remember that I will always love you
with all my heart.
God Bless You Christine.

Part One

As It Was In The Beginning

DAD
1976

It was only four days after mum and dad's twenty-second wedding anniversary, and Auntie Maggie had her lips pressed firmly to my father's as I slipped quietly (my nature), grumpily (adolescence) and more than a little guiltily (Catholicism) down the stairs to breakfast. It was enrolment day for the psychology degree I had chosen against my father's will. The reassuring prospect of bacon, eggs, toast and coffee floated through my mind as my mother rhythmically thumped my father on the chest, pausing only for her sister to return her mouth to his. They were breathing heavily on this hot summer morning.

Orange juice was the sole thought on my mind as I reached the landing, to find my appetite assaulted by an acid scene etching itself onto my psyche. I saw my father unmoving in his sweat-soaked jogging clothes. Death's quarry, he was fast becoming one with the cold unyielding quarry tiles of our porch. He looked like a boxer who had taken a ten count and failed to stir, leaving the crowd suddenly shocked out of their exhilaration and with a disturbing fascinated fear in the pit of their stomachs. I was that crowd. My aunt and my mother acted as referee and coach, kneeling over the supine inanimate fighter – my father.

Everything went pale, then white inside my head. Quiet. I felt I'd seen something I should never have seen; I could come to know something I was not supposed to know. Cold. I felt dead. It wasn't so bad, being dead.

Then it all started coming back, life retrieving itself, demanding me. It poured back into me in unwanted sounds, smells, colours, heat, a light breeze, my father. And my thoughts returned to me like sewage rising out of blocked drains.

My mother saw me out of the corner of her eye and looked up, stricken. I could neither think nor move, a bystander at the scene with no right to be there, little more than a vague outline of character: quiet, frightened, guilty. I fumbled for a thought to connect to, to indulge in, anything but what I was faced with. I was suddenly appalled that it was not my mother pressed to my father's lips, but my aunt. Surely they could, no, *should* be the other way around. Surely these things were still important to us, the most important things to us. What on earth did Maggie think she was doing? And what the hell, for that matter, did *dad* think he was doing?

'I've called the ambulance,' my mother said in a voice so bereft of life that I immediately felt that everyone in the scene was now dead. All of us. 'Go out to the gate and wait for it,' she said and turned back to the remains.

I wanted to help. I wanted to be good and do the right thing, but I headed in the opposite direction; back into the familial house, trying to beat a hasty retreat into a past that had been unfairly and ferociously ripped from my hands. I was scared and confused and alone. It was hard to breathe without crying. It was criminal to be alive. It should be me, dead outside. No! Nobody's dead. I don't know that he's dead. And I would know, believe me, I'd be free and happy and people would have to clear the runway because I'd be taking off.

In front of me waited a brother and a sister, little, looking up to me, worried. They wanted to know what was going on out front. Mark was eight and Elizabeth ten, the two youngest. For some reason one of them took my hand, and the other, seeing this, walked around me and took my other hand. And not knowing why, I walked them out to the front door. I can't explain this. Maybe it was the right thing to do. My body did it, and so I just had to go along with it. Mark, me, Elizabeth; eight, seventeen, ten.

We went to the landing and watched the repeating scene, *breath breath breath heart heart heart*. Mum, dad, Maggie; forty-five, forty-seven, fifty. My brother and sister began to cry. Quietly, rhythmically, their chests heaved with their father's. They seemed to know something I was trying very hard not to know. Kids were like that. We just stood there, holding hands. That's what you're supposed to do, isn't it: hold hands and stick together? We may have stood there for a minute, maybe half an hour; there was no way of telling, time had absconded after putting an end to my father. And I knew it was my fault. I didn't even have to think it up, it was in me already, just waiting to be unwrapped: a soggy heavy indigestible non-refundable Big Mac of guilt.

My 'father'. My last engagement – in the military rather than the romantic sense – with the man had been the usual fission of cold bewildered rigidity on his part and a boiling tearful incredulity on mine. By his look he told me I had been put together wrongly and that there was an end to it: I could not be salvaged from the disgrace that was me. By his word he bid me be no more than a sapling tree espaliered along the brick wall of his being. Yet I loved him, and I needed him. I needed him, just *once*, to put his hand warmly on my shoulder and say, 'Paul, don't worry, you're doing fine. You're OK and I love you.' Just once would have been enough.

But oh, how I hated him. Everywhere, I hated him. There was the one where he had come home from work, hit the trip wire and been blown into bloody bags of bone and guts smashed across the front of the house. Or the one where everyone he knew was there and he said something and I just dismantled him with my wit and wisdom, him crying as he ran out of the room (that, of course, had been me). Or the one where he lets me hit a golf ball instead of just hauling his clubs around for him and I hit a hole-in-one so he lets me play on and I am about to break the course record on the 18th and the whole club house is out now watching from the bar – the 19th hole ha ha ha yup good one dad – and I take the putter and line up the sort of putt I had been making easily all day and I swing that sucker back and bang that hard old golf ball right through my old man's brain and there's the trial and the electric chair and I'm just laughing all the way. I hated him everywhere. Reality wasn't big enough for my fear and hatred, it just couldn't contain it all.

Now it dawned on me that my mother and aunt were not going to stop until the ambulance arrived. I wanted them to leave him alone. I didn't want him back. I knew I should want him back and I knew I did not. I felt I should have taken over from them, that it would have been good form. But I couldn't move any closer than a few feet from the horrifying bodies and the shocking practice they were all involved in. Great slabs of hope for myself had begun to slide off me, like a glacier collapsing into a warmer sea.

What seemed to be hours later – days later – an ambulance quietly pulled up outside, yet broadcasted through livery and lights that there was something extraordinary to be seen nearby. Two paramedics came through the front gate, not too fast and not too slow; not too grim, not too casual. They took over, professional, well drilled. They had a studied reverence and efficiency about them, yet were clearly unimpressed by so mundane an end. I couldn't look at them, these able men. I didn't like them for coming and knowing exactly what to do. My father didn't teach me anything that would make me stronger. I went back inside again but everywhere was my father. I stood still for a while, staring at the carpet, then turned around and went back to the porch. I knew I was supposed to be on the porch.

Apologetically the paramedics moved my father to the lawn after trying to resuscitate him for a while, a while that failed dismally to give the impression that they had tried long enough. Dad lay on the warm grass, withering in the heat. *All flesh is as grass*. But at least they left him alone, gave him some peace, a quiet time to himself to mull things over, to reflect on whether this was really what he had intended at so prosperous a time in his and our young lives. He had six children.

The people gathered there that morning stared at his body, then at each other, at the ground, back at him, around and around the mulberry bush, we all fall down. The silence deepened, imposing itself over the garden like water, submerging me with the others. The weight of it pressed down heavily, and in this ocean of quiet I could not speak, and could hear nothing but the rhythmic thump, thump of my heart like the engine of an overhead boat. But I knew they would find me down there. They would be relentless and they would know my soul and they would find me and punish me. I had ruined everything, and I would not get away with it. In that house I didn't even get away with things I hadn't done: a sin in mind is a sin in deed. Beyond the garden's perimeters hurried a moving background of leaves and pedestrians and traffic that seemed to have politely muffled their usual noise out of respect for the solemnity of the occasion. A pedestrian on his way to the local shops caught a glimpse of the cadaver and looked a little too long and obviously, only to wrench his face away as he realised that he too was being stared at, from the porch. Having got what he wanted, more than he had dreamed of, he accelerated away, ashamed, fascinated.

And I too had got more than I had wanted, more than I had dreamed of. The previous night I had committed to the Gods my usual ritual of the time: a prayer for my father's early demise. That I had suddenly been granted so emphatic and categorical a response left me singularly surprised, alarmed and culpable. They would find me and they would punish me.

'Paul.' My mother's voice from far off.

'Paul.' The name reached down and hauled me back up and I broke through to the surface. And it was still all happening. 'Will you go to get Mary from work?' my mother said. 'I want you to get her home without telling her what's happened.'

I said 'OK' and went back inside to ring my girlfriend's parents to ask for their help.

'Hi,' I said. I felt a bit stuck then, but something inside me didn't and it just kept going: 'Look, I don't know how to say this so I'll just have to blurt it out. My father has just died, at home, out on the front steps.'

'Oh, Paul,' the phone said. It was as if there was no person at the other end, and yet at the same time I'd never felt so close to anyone.

'Yes,' I said flatly. 'And I need to go and get one of my sisters. Can you help me out?'

They drove me to Mary. It was strange being in that car, out in the rapid important world where no one knew. As soon as Mary saw me, the beginning of distress impressed itself on her sixteen-year-old face and I realised my mother's plan was already undone.

'Dad's not well,' I said. Mary just looked at me, huge worried bovine eyes, waiting. Her eyes said, gently, *Why do you lie to us, and on a day that is going to be so unbearable?*

Helplessly and hopelessly out of my depth, I couldn't see how on earth my mother thought I was going to manage to get Mary home without telling her anything. But then, how could my mother think at all right now. If she could, that would not be right, would it? I was freezing up, my mind temporarily out of use – please try again later, sorry for any inconvenience.

Kind Selwyn, my girlfriend's father, turned around and gently said, 'You're going to have to tell her, Paul.' Oh how I loved Selwyn in that moment – if he knew this, then perhaps he could one day tell me *everything*.

'Mary, I've got some really bad news.' Pause, swallow, but I couldn't swallow, as my saliva had evacuated with my mind. 'Dad died this morning. At home.'

The appalling shock first entered her eyes, and then flooded her face to flow down and through her and into us both. She leaned in to me and began to sob, that young girl in her uniform, my sister, my little sister. She didn't know just how fragile was the support offered her by her piteously unprepared brother. I struggled for what to do in order not to totally collapse. I knew I had to be strong, but I did not really know what that was. I had after all managed to tell her the truth, and although it wasn't poetry, at least it wasn't from a stranger. I found this thought consoling, and I let go in myself a little, subsided slightly inside. Mary and I huddled in the back seat of the car, hiding from the fierce world outside, heading home, always home.

We arrived to a crowd of bewildered beings, not a seat left in the house, a sell-out. How on earth had they all heard? And come so quickly? It was frightening. I was caught up in something smothering, sucking the life out of everything. I walked into the lounge reddening with anger and embarrassment, and as I veered towards a chair, it instantly emptied itself of its incumbent. I was stunned as I felt the first full flush of the power bestowed by the ashamedly alive on the mourner. As the living maintained a dutiful and cautious distance, I felt both totally exposed and utterly alone. This, it seemed to me, was not new.

I stood up. I could feel it in their minds: 'Paul has stood up. He is standing alone by that chair. Should I go over to him? Does he want to be left alone? Would it be wrong to give him a nod? A smile? Or wrong not to? No-one else is moving . . .' Everyone in the room noticed I had stood up. Wasn't this exactly, precisely what I had always wanted? I was appalled at myself.

Out of the front door I fled, away from my terrible neediness, over the porch where dad had crashed. I went down the side of the house and leant against the wall to stare at the grass he had made me mow every Saturday, whether or not it needed it. Maybe he knew in his bones he would be laid out upon it one fine morning, and wanted it just so.

His body was gone. *He* was gone. He was 'a gonner'. I had not seen him being taken away; it must have happened while I was in the car with Mary. I wondered what it had been like for my mother to see him, indestructible, carried away, forever. He often got carried away. He was a human dynamo and would extract every ounce of pace and life from each stutter of the second hand, and then one day – today – *tick tick* **TOCK!** Dead.

My mind fled once more, out of the garden, beyond the endless stretch of clouds, beyond the darkness of my father. But then, *Bling*! Auntie Maggie suddenly appeared in front of me – an obese needy angel. As a boy I had been there one morning when her girth was measured: 52 inches. I couldn't believe it. When everyone had left I picked up the cloth tape measure and held it up; 52 inches was over my head. From then on whenever I looked at Auntie Maggie I could not help thinking about being wrapped around her stomach, not tall enough to reach all the way. I wondered if she would expand faster than I would grow tall.

There she was, in her fullness, having long ago left the adjective 'plump' in her wake. To my utter astonishment I heard myself splutter out, 'I love you, Maggie.' How had she done that? It was a trick. Somehow she had just reached in and pulled it out of me. I immediately wanted to withdraw the declaration and myself with it, but she grabbed me, clutched me to her huge bosom. I was shocked at what I had said. I didn't love her at all. She held me, held me, it was like being held under water. Only after a week-long minute did she pull back, a little, but she did not release me from this new suffocating intimacy.

Through tears of relief she said, 'At least one good thing has come out of all this, Paul.' I couldn't believe my ears. Jesus H. Christ! It wasn't right. I just knew it wasn't right, it wasn't the sort of thing anyone should be saying to me. I had to find a way out and somehow I understood the currency – I knew I had to give her one more hug to be free. I closed myself down even more, and I opened my arms, and I did it. I felt nauseous and giddy. Don't faint. Do not faint now, mate! Even at seventeen years of age my arms would not contain her girth. She was a jumbo capital O in my little parenthesis. But I earned my release and walked around the house, away from Maggie. As soon as I reached the front door again, the porch, I found myself walking up the steps and back into the house and the lounge full of laughing Irishmen who had taken over my mourning.

My father had died the morning after my mother had found a condom on the floor outside my bedroom, and I had felt damned in that particular and extraordinary way Catholics are trained for from birth. I had lied to my mother and skulked to bed that evening working and reworking my story for its next airing, which would undoubtedly involve my father. He was sharp as a tack, all critical faculties present and accounted for. My story was weak and I could not count on my producing tears again. My father's death had saved me from an uncomfortable grilling, and for that I was truly grateful, Amen. Perhaps, for me, that was the 'one good thing' that had 'come out of all this'. I was worse than Maggie. Much worse.

But because of that condom, I'd been left with a certainty of what he must have been thinking about immediately before, possibly during his heart attack. Sitting there on the steps, panting and sweating, he would have been thinking about his Catholic boy having carnal knowledge of a Catholic girl. And then it was obvious. I didn't even need to think about it, it was hard-wired into me: it was this state of affairs, as it were, that had driven his blood pressure beyond what his dairy-product-and-cigarette-laden system could endure. It was all very Oedipal, and the thoughts that had begun tormenting me in the hostile courtroom of my mind were rapidly compli-cating and conflicting. I had ruined everything. This is what I do: I ruin everything. And I would have to pay for the rest of my life. And then they will find me, the angels, and they will know me, and they will take me to Hell.

As he had been a big fish, my father's funeral was a substantial enterprise, streets blocked off by police motorcycles, mourners spilling outside the church and onto the sports field next door. I could not believe that all these people had actually liked my father, and assumed it was a welcome and rather fortuitous day off for all in the firm. I later discovered I was quite wrong: these people, and most especially the labourers, had experienced a warmth and civility from my father I had never known.

The funeral was everything I had tried not to want and everything I hated myself for wanting. *Everyone* was looking at us, that poor McDermott family, mum and her six Catholic children, three of us altar-boys in this very church. They were trying not to look at us, but just *had* to, to see what this much pain looked like when it was all put together and dressed in three suits and four dresses and given some valium and a stiff sherry. They were looking at me. Did they feel sorry for me, pity me? And the girls my age – did this look attractive? And when I felt the weight of my father through the brass handles of the coffin pressing into my palm – did I look strong, able to cope with *anything*, a brave young man? Not, hopefully, a relieved young man.

Out into the sunshine, lowering the coffin clumsily into the hearse. Was that a thump I heard? Had dad rolled onto his side? And the rollers in the hearse – of course, rollers! Why hadn't I been expecting rollers? *What* was I thinking about? But those rollers, what a cool idea. I wondered what they did before rollers. Then backing off, backing away, onto the sports field to stand alone, to be noticed, pitied. I could not stop myself wanting to drink it in.

The black car ride. Not a sound. Not a vibration. People pulling over and pedestrians stopping on the pavement, out of respect, to look. Then out into the sun again. I was feeling sick. The heat, the neediness, the gluttonous feasting on my father's death. A huge hole, big enough for a small car, and a pile of dirt covered in fake grass matting. Who did they think they were kidding with that? A handful of dirt given to me. Pause. They were all looking at me. They didn't know what I would have given to throw this at him while he was still alive.

I watched the dirt fall from my hand onto his coffin. I watched my revenge, and heard it hit the shining wooden lid, *thud shhishhhh*. Only the best for dad. But I had my revenge, it coursed through my veins and breathed in and out of me, for I had out-lived him.

Backing away, back, back. It all went white, like an over-exposed photograph.

TOM
14 October 1993

I waited in anxious silence outside the house of someone whose death had come alive in them. I sat in my little car, pretending I was fine and relaxed and that nothing phased me. I liked to give the impression, even to myself, that I was not still a mess inside. I waited on the side of a road that curved away before and behind me just as it was designed to in the town planning office. I was confronted by a profound sense of barrenness, inside and out. This street and I, we were not a part of life at all, we were on a stage. No other cars cluttered the side of the road; they all had their own pre-planned little driveways and garages. No children played on the streets, no dogs dared bark, no pedestrians ruined the effect by venturing out on the pavements. Not even the trees seemed to stir. Nothing moved, nothing made a sound. The houses seemed to be holding back, listening. It would not have been out of place if a tumble-weed had rolled down the road accompanied by the lament of a single quavering note from a mouth organ. Except this was an autumnal England.

The property belonged to an elderly woman who lived anonymously, and acrimoniously, in this small military town.

The house was a modest 1950s semi-detached, mirrored and repeated out of sight in both directions: plain, uninteresting, indicating by its very design that nothing of any significance was meant to happen within its four walls. Yet I awaited my appointment with her dreading and hoping all. My gut felt cold and empty. What on earth was I *do*ing there?

As I sat sweaty-palmed in my car I began to regret being involved with the hospice charity at all, feeling a vague nostalgia for the 9-to-5 security of the 1980s: wake up = radio STRAIGHT on in case I was immediately confronted by one of my own thoughts; wash = radio on louder; eat = news on the radio and a newspaper and 'Thought for the Day' in case another one of mine slipped through the net; the underground = walkman playing something I thought would impress the sort of woman I would want to impress if she asked to listen (which she never did); the International Stock Exchange = computer screens and meetings and documents and meetings; a workout at the gym = eye-level MTV with dancing girls who were not interested in what was on my walkman; home = television; bed = racked by paranoia and self-loathing and every little interaction of the day scraping painfully across the rasp of my ego as I searched forensically for criticism or blunder.

A district nurse pulled up in front of me in her own little car. You could feel the twitching curtains along the road. She interrupted my paranoid reverie by introducing herself, but I was so distracted that I missed her name entirely. I moved with her towards the ominous little house now not only anxious but also slightly disoriented. Death was in there, and

I wanted to face it, again, face something definite. I had already realised that if I wanted to truly understand something, I had to stand right in front of it, all by myself.

We crossed the road in an awkward silence. I didn't feel so good, and suddenly I was desperate for a pee. 'A deep breath and a leap,' whispered Goethe as I arrived at the front door, a door that would become as familiar to me as my own. I rang the bell and a submerged figure appeared beyond the watery glass. Like water tends to do, the distortions of the glass made whoever was behind it look very short and stocky. The door opened and there the old woman stood, proudly erect at five foot, barrel-round. She grinned broadly at the nurse, glanced at me in a pleasant but cursory fashion and indicated, by walking off, that we should follow her inside.

I sat when invited on a huge sofa and stared nervously around a room so valiantly decorated it increased my growing unease. The ceiling hung low, covered with dirty polyurethane rectangles full of tiny holes like a battalion of factory-made rain clouds. Cornicing was glued around the edges to keep the clouds in the room, drifting only eight feet above a typhonic swirl of pattern and colours: Gaudian wallpaper hung heroically over Daliesque carpet. There were dark laminate cabinets, the colossal fake velvet sofa with matching chairs, and sitting mightily against the wall the brooding ever-watchful television set. I thought rather irreverently that I too would be seriously ill if I had to live in that dense kaleidoscopic frenzy.

The room conveyed the sense of a life defined, referenced and shelved; an impression that little had actually happened other than the gradual accumulation of this flotsam and jetsam. Perhaps I was just one more piece. Yet each small object had some self-importance about it, much like the woman I had come to visit. And there sat I, about to be born into her world, before she could no longer tell anyone about it, before she went completely cold and was burned to dust in a furnace.

By now feeling seasick, I was horrified when the nurse suddenly stood to leave. I stood with her and smiled weakly, torn out of my interior's delirium by the look of pity and hope that flickered across her eyes. As I sat down again to stare at the veneer coffee table that pressed urgently against my knees, I felt alone and exposed in a way that felt familiar. I had been cast out upon some vast ocean with neither map nor compass, needing to learn how to navigate by the stars alone. It felt dreadful. It was perfect.

What if I stood up and said 'I've just got to see a man about a dog.' And before she knew it I'd be out the front door and into my car and off down the road? I'd drive all the way to southern France, and live off my credit cards. In summer I would press grapes with my bare feet with French girls with their full black skirts pulled up over long brown legs. I would slowly learn the language. And fall in love with a dark-eyed, dark-haired young woman, slight over-bite, perfect little breasts, and we would marry and have children. Then there would be this huge flood and I'd save the young and the elderly and everyone in the village would love me. 'Tea?!'

I followed her into the kitchen like an unmoored boat drifting with whatever tide the moon exerted. From the kitchen

I got another angle on the garden that was visible through aluminium sliding doors at the end of the lounge. The garden was rectangles, flanked on the right by a dead straight concrete path. There was a contained rectangle of grass, a rectangle of vegetable garden, and two rectangles of stone paving, one by the sliding doors and one at the far end, which ended in a vertical green rectangle of hedge.

She saw me staring out at the parade of garden and, as if reading my mind, said, 'Tom was in the military.'

'Ah,' I said, in perfect French.

We returned to the lounge and sat, tea in hand, at opposite ends of the consuming sofa. She told me about receiving her death sentence, and finished her monologue with 'But at least I had Tom.' She went on to tell me that one month after she had been diagnosed, her husband of forty-eight years had also received a diagnosis of cancer. At least his prognosis had been better than hers, which meant that he would be there to look after her until she died. But he had not managed this. Tom had died within a month of being diagnosed. He had died emptying his bowels on their bed upstairs.

Val had sat at his side bewildered and frightened, as I now sat at hers. Suddenly she was not only dying but acutely *aware* that she was dying. She thought in those Arctic moments that it was she who was supposed to die first, and that he was supposed to be there looking after her. She had looked at her husband, dead on their bed, and thought to herself, now strangely alone in the room, 'This will happen to me.'

That was where I came in.

Val was seventy-four when we met, and although it is a bit rude to say so, she looked all of it. If you have seen the *Star Wars* films, you may remember Yoda, who was clearly based on this woman: a squat, amused, wrinkled being with an air of mischievous awareness and a penetrating stare. That, with a smear of red lipstick, but without the cloak and pointed ears, was Val. The week after my first visit I rang her doorbell and noticed it took her a couple of minutes to swim from the sofa to the glass front door. On surfacing she beamed up at me from the doorway. I looked down smiling, but in my mind went, 'Oh my God, why hadn't I noticed *that* before?' From her gaping mouth protruded three (only) teeth so separated from each other that each appeared to be leading a life entirely independent of the others.

I found myself slightly more immune to the décor, and once offered a seat on the sofa I sank quietly down, and down, as if in quicksand, my arm protruding from the crevice between cushions, then only a hand, then gone, forgotten.

It was not the sort of visit one begins with 'How are you?' because the only honest answer is 'I'm dying. How are you?' So I gave an impression of sitting quietly and calmly that seemed convincing enough for Val to begin talking, which she would always do in her own time and her own way. She idly chatted about the 'news' and the weather and what nurses had visited her until she came to inviting me to share some tea with her. She did this with a delighted affection for the word itself, as if she had by chance stumbled upon this long-sought-after treasure: '*Tea*?!' Big grin. Three teeth.

A photograph of Tom in uniform looked down on me, in more ways than one, from the bookshelf at what was to always be Val's end of the sofa. Tom looked as though he expected to take the lead, to go on ahead. He had.

Not being a fan of English tea – I liked to pretend I had left behind a need for the homely reassurance offered by milky tea for a Zen-like independence – I tried to leave my lukewarm cup without saying anything. I hoped this would go unnoticed. It did not. I didn't want the tea, but I also didn't want to hurt her feelings. On this, my first solo visit, I was to do almost everything wrong. It was to take some recovering from.

'What's wrong with your tea?' Val demanded, looking exasperatedly from the cup to me and back again.

'Just letting it cool down a bit,' I said. Sometimes a lie would just pop right out of me like that, before I knew it was coming, like it was dad on my case and I was in deep trouble. My penance from that time onwards was that she would add so much milk as to make it no longer tea at all, but something more like lukewarm milk that had had a brown crayon dipped into it. 'You like it not so hot, don't you?' she would say. I worked out my karma and drank the 'tea'.

'Another cup?'

Like an idiot I said, 'Yes, if you're making one.'

'Well, it's not about to make itself, is it?'

This time she delivered the tea with the teabag still in the cup and a teaspoon for me to retrieve it but no saucer. I wondered where to put the bag once it was out.

Val appeared to enjoy my shy discomfort, enjoyed being entertained for a change. I was beginning to notice how acutely she was observing me, as if I were a patient possessed by some unknown affliction that she would eventually diagnose and then give me a prescription for.

'You can just leave it on the spoon (pause), but it will go in the rubbish bin under the kitchen sink (pause). That's the compost (pause). I was told you do gardening.' Val was pacing her speech so that an imbecile could understand her. Gardening? I'd had little experience of gardening other than lawn mowing. When I was thirteen, I used to ride my bicycle over to my father's friend's house to water his plants while he was away in Australia. It was a very hot summer, and I used to enjoy standing there with the hose. I would watch the water rainbow over the thick-leaved plants, the reassuringly dense smells of damp earth and wet warm concrete. The kidney stones of my home life seemed to wash away from me, like the gravel that washed out of the plant beds to sluice down the driveway. I would stand there quiet on that hot concrete driveway, thinking about how I would spend the money I was so easily earning.

It was just wonderful. But I didn't get the job again the

next time dad's friend went away, some problem about gravel loss.

'Oh,' was all I managed to say to Val's confusing me with a gardener, but it was I who was confused about why I was there.

She went on, without missing a beat, to give me the facts of her life. She was born Evelyn Turner, with Europe reverberating from the Great War. As a young child she was told that her mother had been a prostitute who had given her up to an orphanage. She remained there until the age of fourteen, the end of the Great Depression. She was adopted by a couple who could not conceive children of their own and, as so often happens upon adopting, the mother immediately fell pregnant with the first of her own children. Val was left in the somewhat unexpected position of having siblings to compete with for love and attention.

The remainder of her adolescence, and in fact the rest of her life, was passed in Aldershot. The town was gearing up for the Second World War when Val applied to the Post Office for a job, where she remained employed until she retired. In 1936 she had met Tom Hall and through him found at last a family, Tom's family, who welcomed her unreservedly and as one of their own. Three years after she met Tom, the Third Reich drew England into war. With Val turning twenty years of age, Tom enlisted in the air force and went off to fight.

Although they were engaged that same year, it was another three years before Tom and Val were married, on April Fool's Day. Ten years later their daughter Christine was born, an experience Val found so physically horrendous that she decided then and there that Christine was to be her only child. This event seemed to confirm to Val what she had suspected for years: that her marriage was the enemy of all that was vital, original and promising.

Val said all of this in a measured, matter-of-fact way, until she suddenly slumped forward and dropped her head toward her lap. She had begun on the story of her life from the time of her daughter's birth, a territory unexplored since the events themselves. She found then and there in her little low room that the power of these memories was such that it could easily buckle her. They pulled her down bodily as well as emotionally, into the quiet resignation that had become the background to her being-in-the-world. Val felt her life had been extinguished at Christine's birth, not as a result of Christine herself but of what being a mother came to mean to Val: the forfeiture of her own biography. To her, all that was possible and hopeful in her life had been scuppered. She saw ahead only a predictable posthumous pedestrianism. Her life was to become uniform, not unlike her garden – trimmed, fenced, concreted over where deemed prudent.

'And I didn't like it,' she said. 'I never liked it. I just did it because I felt I had to.' She sobbed and leaned forward, her head in her hands, her elbows resting on her knees. This was not what I had been expecting. I tried to beam rays of Empathy and Congruence and Unconditional Positive Regard at her, because that was what I had been trained to do. Inside I was beginning to flounder.

'I think sometimes I should just have let him go with that

woman,' she said into her palms. 'I don't think he ever forgave me for that.'

What woman? Had she talked about a woman? How could I have missed that?

We were sitting at separate ends of her sofa. I wanted to help. It was terrible what I did, crushing: I slid along the sofa, without being invited, and put my arm around Val's shoulders. It was in the Manual, Chapter 2, Hugs and Tissues. She sat bolt upright, immobilised and tense. The sobbing stopped, immediately, possibly permanently. I was left in the embarrassing position of sitting there with my arm draped around her like she was my girlfriend, the used teabag discarded on the table. I suddenly had a craving to run. As I tried to surreptitiously withdraw the offending arm, she glanced up at me. I saw in her face years of pent-up anguish, dammed up once more against an unreceptive world. I was that world.

'Sorry about that,' she said. Those should have been my words: *'No, Val, give yourself a break, it was me. I've been trained to do that sort of terrible stuff to people. I am an abomination.'*

'I don't know what came over me,' she said, painfully, for both of us. And I let her. 'It must be the steroids.' She stared into a familiar abyss of lost opportunities.

'I'll make us a cup of tea,' she said as she pulled herself up and out of the depths of the sofa and memory. She slowly made her way back to her kitchen, defeated. Frozen to my seat, appalled at what I had done, I couldn't budge. Inside I shouted at myself, 'Bugger! Bugger! You stupid bugger!'

I might as well have leaned over and punched her when she had begun to cry. *Thwack!* 'Pull yourself together, woman! Worse things happen at sea!'

On Val's return from the kitchen, the glacial void I had engineered echoed with polite, empty conversation. She said, 'I went . . .'

'Oh, did you?'

'Yes, it was lovely and . . .'

'Sounds nice.'

'Did you see that programme on . . . ?'

'No, I missed it.'

'It was all about . . .'

'Really.'

'Yes, and . . .'

'Mmmm.'

'Still, you must be very busy today.'

'—'

'You've got all your hospice work and things.'

'—'

'Don't let me keep you.'

When I left Val didn't look at me. I was hoping for some look or word of reassurance. Everything was the wrong way around. Quite rightly, no quarter was given. I left her that day feeling worse than useless: I was an impediment.

When I returned the following week, we resumed what became our usual places on the sofa. But now there was a pile of magazines over a foot tall between us. The Wall. Neither Val nor I mentioned its presence. It was the Iron Curtain, it was Cold War Berlin in that little room. It was humiliating and intimidating, but this time for the appropriate person. Rooted into that sofa – Val, the magazines, and I – like her three disparate teeth, we were ostensibly united in purpose, yet were already separated by a seemingly unbridgeable breech.

A HOLE IN THE GROUND
November 1993

Thursday tended to be the day I sat through committee meetings, ran training sessions, supervised volunteers. I'd become involved with the hospice charity at the beginning of the year, when I heard about its plan to offer support to people with a life-threatening illness to remain at home with the familiar for as long as possible. After a few months I became Director of Training and Development. I guess they could see I knew I had a lot to learn, so would make the ideal teacher.

Thursday was also the day I usually saw Val. I sat down when invited and left when she hinted, in broad brush strokes, that it was time for me to be gone. In all other ways there were no rules, no map, no recipe; it was the experience itself that pulled us forward, bound only by the laws of gravity and time.

'Do you know what I've got?' Val asked, eyes sparkling and eyebrows raised, thrilled at the chance to put me on the spot.

I shook my head, 'No, I don't, Val.'

'Or how long then?'

'No,' I said.

'Myeloma,' she said. 'Do you know what that is?'

'Some sort of cancer,' I said, but I couldn't even spell *my low ma*. It was like my first therapy patient, I couldn't spell skits oh frenick either. Maybe that's what cured him. I liked to think so.

'It's cancer of the blood and bone,' Val said matter-of-factly. The significance of this was immediately clear: how do you rid yourself of a cancer that is in your very blood and bone? I was glad it was not me with the my low ma. But I wasn't glad it was her.

'When the doctor told me, I couldn't believe it,' she said. 'I thought he must have confused me with someone else. I mean, I knew I'd have to go some day, but I wasn't ready for anything like this. And then to be told that I would only have a couple of months, possibly three, just like that!' She tried to click her fingers but couldn't, and it clearly irritated her. 'I couldn't believe it. Still can't sometimes.'

I asked Val to tell me everything she knew about my low ma, so that in a small way we could begin to occupy some similar understanding, to put some stakes in the ground. I had not understood that the ground itself would be constantly moving, separating, dividing, like the cancer itself.

She talked about her myeloma with curiosity and relief, relief at being able to talk about it without hearing a response like, 'I'm sure you'll pull through' or 'Best not talk about it, don't you think?' or 'How about a nice cup of tea?' or 'Did I tell you about So-and-so? They thought she was at death's door but she's leaping around like a gazelle now!'

Our conversation went in and out of cancer and gardening

and dying and tea and death and the neighbours, until Val leant forward on the sofa, her loose-skinned forearms resting on her floralled thighs, and stared out through the lounge into the quiet garden.

'What's that on the lawn?' I asked, following her gaze out to a pale, curvaceous structure, forlorn on the grass.

'It's a pond. A fish pond,' she said, with a raise of an eyebrow as she leaned back and turned to inspect me. I'd taken the bait.

'And what do you plan to do with it?' I said, my eyes fixed on the albino sea-lion marooned on this suburban lawn.

'Put it in the ground, of course!' She looked at me doubtfully, as though my intellect was in the something-wriggling-in-a-primordial-pond category.

'How long has it been lying there?' I said calmly, resolute. I would not be hurt or insulted. I'd had a lifetime's practice at this.

'I ordered it when I was told about the cancer – mine, not Tom's – and it's been sitting there ever since. It was going to be the last thing to be put into the garden, before it got too bad,' she said, turning back to the stillness outdoors. 'You know.'

But of course I didn't know, and nor did she. That was a large part of the problem, not knowing what 'it' would be like when 'it' got worse. And worse again after that, and then worse still, until 'It' was as bad as 'It' could be without Val being dead. What was 'IT' going to do to her physically and emotionally and mentally, and how would that in turn affect her physically and emotionally and mentally and spiritually? And so on and so on, deeper and deeper into her.

'Now I can't get down on my knees to do what needs to be done,' she said, unwittingly describing what her future would require of the both of us. With clenched fists she said, 'It's so frus*trat*ing! I can't bear to be useless.' There was a long pause as we both stared out to the garden as if it were some inaccessible province, now beyond Val's footfall.

'You're a gardener, aren't you? That's what I'm told,' she said hopefully again.

'I don't know who could have told you that,' I said, only then realising it would have been either Irene or Anna, two of the nurses I knew from the charity who attended to Val. It was clever and kind of them to put such a practical idea into her mind.

'Never mind. Lying, were they?' Val said.

She turned away from me and in doing so gave me the distinct impression that I had turned away from her. But then something inside of me spoke out loud; it might have been me, 'Well, I'm not really a gardener,' it said. 'But if you tell me what to do I'm willing to give it a go. It's up to you.' Of course it was; it had to be up to her, in the end.

Val beamed at me, then returned her gaze to the pond. 'It's fibreglass.'

'Ah.' I knew quite a bit about fibreglass. Having surfed in the southern hemisphere for years, I had spent many an evening repairing my surfboard with epoxy resin and fibreglass matting, getting a high and nauseous on the fumes. When I remember surfing I can still feel my body undulating over the swell as I sit on my board, waiting, buoyed by the rhythm of the endless waves. Waiting.

Like an old sunken ship resurfacing into the world, Val rose from her end of the sofa. Upon righting herself she listed to starboard to look down at me and by raising an eyebrow signalled I should follow in her wake, slowly, patiently.

She sedately cruised to a side-cupboard drawer to salvage a single key, and made slow headway over to the French doors at the end of the lounge. I followed quietly, a little tense and expectant. She unlocked the doors, carefully, deliberately, making it clear to me that I was to do what is so importantly conveyed to us as children: look!

This was how Val passed on to me the idiosyncrasies and practices of the contained religion of her home: a slow deliberate demonstration with a knowing smile on her face, as though she were unlocking doors to the mysterious powers of the ancients. And of course the ritual was appropriate; this was *her world* she was opening to me, the secrets and memories and experiences of a life soon to be snuffed out. This passing on of the rites would in turn confer on me responsibilities and powers no one else may have had in relation to her at any time. And I could use this position for or against her, as she weakened and deteriorated towards her seemingly already writ conclusion. Perhaps for Val the conclusion would come to just one further question, *the* question. As if she was already in training, it was rare to find her without a magazine of brainteasers and crosswords in her hands. The wall of magazines that lay between us was almost entirely made up of puzzles: solvable but legion.

Val led me out to a cold inhospitable day. She breathed heavily at the effort of moving a mere twenty yards. On reaching the pond she unceremoniously kicked it, but trembled at this more than the pond did. What was I going to do if she fell over and had a heart attack or something? My father's death, it was there, in the garden with me.

After she'd regained her breath and both of us our balance, Val tugged me over to the rear of the garden, to the brigade of flowerbeds as it would be in spring. There in the centre was a parade square of soil, surrounded by broken rectangular paving, headstones of what had been before.

Pointing to the ground she said 'Here', as if this was to be the very plot in which she would be buried, 'with the small end pointing towards the house.' I wondered which was her 'small end'.

'Fine,' I said, nervous and uncomfortable. I would help. I would not be nothing.

With a military nod Val said, 'We'll start next week, if the ground isn't already too hard, and if there's nothing else I want you to do.' She looked up at me to hold my gaze for that telling split second longer than normal, letting me know I had been engaged beyond the social niceties. Before trundling slowly back to the house, she smiled at me, almost warmly.

SHOPPING
December 1993

The committee smiled at me too, almost warmly, as they sat encircling a small herd of tables. The meetings were held early on Thursday afternoons, in a tension brought about by the juxtaposition of a palpable underlying hostility and overbearing niceness. Afterwards I would drive over to Val's and try to leave all of the unpleasantness behind. I wanted to concentrate on what was of utmost importance: a patient, a person, Val.

I arrived at Val's without my gardening clothes – the pond would have to wait until spring as the ground was already cold and hardening. It did not seem likely to me that Val would be buried this winter either, as two months after meeting her she was already beyond her prognosis and going strong. I wanted to believe this was because of me. That my devotion and compassion meant that Val's cancer had miraculously gone into remission, her life now flushed with meaning. I didn't really believe any of this, not really. But then again, maybe I did.

On the other hand, her persistence left me in a bit of a predicament, because I was due to go off to the other side of the world for five weeks over Christmas. When I had signed up for this, I had not expected her to live that long. Timidly I told Val this – not the bit about expecting her to be dead by now – and all she said was, 'I'll see you when you get back then. If you want to come.'

'Yup, I'll want to come,' I said, wondering if she could still be alive by February. But she had nothing further to say on the matter. Subject closed. The following Christmas would be a very different sort of leaving altogether. But this visit was like many that were to follow, week after week, broken only by my travels: I sat in her lounge, beyond the magazines, and for this I received an ever-developing narration of her history. Her past was like a photographic plate she would leave in the solution a bit longer, just a bit more, as little details appeared, were exposed. Details that were always in there, but had remained hidden. Timing is everything. She was trying to come to terms with her life so she would be able to come to terms with dying. She had a backlog. She was not alone in this. Val seemed to need a witness, and so I began to feel necessary and somehow significant. Then out of the blue she cancelled the next visit. When I did finally get to see her again, I learnt much more about my place in the scheme of things.

On arriving, I parked in the driveway. Val had told me it was OK to leave my car there now, because she could not see hers leaving her garage again in her lifetime. I climbed out of my little VW and when I pressed Val's doorbell I heard the ding-dong clearly from inside. The volume on that thing must have been on maximum. I waited. I had been waiting two weeks to see her.

Nothing.

Not a sound.

Feeling conspicuous and uncomfortable, I looked up and down the street. There was no-one around. I was feeling a little guilty, as usual. Perhaps the whole neighbourhood knew that I was the guy who had stopped that elderly dying woman from crying. *There he is, boys, get him!!*

I rang the doorbell again. I waited.

Nothing.

Not a sound.

It was cold out, and I shook my watch even though I could see the second hand was moving. It was working fine. I was sure I was doing something wrong, I just could not figure out what it was. I went back to the car and checked the dashboard clock, one-forty-eight. I had arrived about fifteen minutes early. My solar plexus began to tighten. Something bad was happening. Was it only inside me, this bad thing, or was it happening outside? I couldn't tell. My childhood was like that.

From my first visit I knew the front door would not be locked, but instead I chose the alley between the garage and the house that led along to the backyard. The bolt was stiff and cold when I put my hand through the hole in the gate to slide it free. It gave way with a stentorian complaint, loud enough to wake the dead.

Down along the path and out to the back garden, my mind became strangely empty and still, my stomach knotted. I turned left and moved anxiously towards the glass sliding doors at the far end of the lounge. There was a pale blue flickering light coming from inside. Angels, fairies from the garden. I pressed my face to the pane like some cheeky kid in a passing car, and there was Val, as large as life, collapsed in her chair. She was immobilised in front of the massive television set that had robbed her of so much.

Val was dead, I knew it. As I raised my hand to the door handle, my heart skipped a beat when she suddenly shuffled in her chair, in response, I assumed, to something on the television that had literally moved her.

It was both a shock and an anti-climax, one I was both grateful for and annoyed by. I knew then that she had heard the doorbell on that cold afternoon, but would be having none of it until the designated hour. I was getting to know my place, and it was a lowly place. I didn't have a white steed, or a suit of shining armour, or a beautiful princess to be rescued; I had a banged up old car and wore someone else's clothes and was faced with a fire-breathing dragon.

I returned to my old car and started the engine to get the heater going. I felt like driving off, punishing her for not shaping her life around my goodness, for not being defined by my righteousness. As I sat there, superfluous, I understood that I was being scheduled in between soaps, in by two and out by five. 'OK', I thought to myself, 'this is how it's going to be.'

On the way to the front door at two o'clock, I decided not to bother with the doorbell. I just waited. I could hear theme music issuing from the lounge as the credits rolled, endlessly acknowledging anyone remotely involved in the soap opera. Once the accolades and plaudits were spent, Val drifted up to the glass door. She greeted me with a broad grin, broader than usual, even though she was getting no credits, no recognition – she was in the wrong business. Maybe I was too, if applause was what I was interested in.

She had trundled up with a shopping trolley lined with a large white plastic rubbish bag. The bag contained a shovel, its wooden handle broken. Like my grand-father, Pop, Val came from a time where a thing that was broken was still of use, still somehow essential.

Val moved to one side for me to go in, then pushed the shopping trolley outside and closed the door. She followed me indoors and, breaking the routine of tea, went knees first onto the sofa to 'case the joint' across the road. She peeked through the net curtains at the large inviting pile of wet sand outside the hushed house opposite. It was, apparently, just the sort of sand 'we' needed to make a base in the earth for the pond.

'School is still in, so we have about an hour,' she said. Joining her on the sofa and lifting a corner of the net curtain, I suddenly felt part of the community. I saw there was no foot traffic and guessed there was little chance of road traffic. I had gathered Val's plan was something a little more skulduggerous than my going over and just *asking* for some sand.

Nodding towards the house opposite, she said, 'Gone away,' in the clipped grammar of the agent provocateur. Nosy neighbours were the only obvious hazard. I received my instructions. It was as though Val had a gun pointed at my head and was making me do this; I just couldn't see the gun. I could feel it. Otherwise surely I would have just said, 'No. Let's jump into the car and drive up to the garden centre and buy some sand.'

I took the shopping trolley and hit the path at a good clip, but slowed at the road to appear casual. I casually crossed the road, casually pulled out the broken shovel, casually stole the sand. It did that great thing that sand does in the rain – it was only wet about ¼ of an inch in, under that it was perfectly dry as if it were in the desert where it hadn't rained for a million years. I liked that, that underneath things can be totally different.

I looked over to Val's house and saw her face peering out from the bottom corner of the front window. On seeing me looking she let the curtain drop. Why was she hiding from me? Perhaps it was just a reflex. Or had she seen someone coming? The road was empty, shiny wet with drizzle. Maybe she had seen that the house I was stealing from wasn't empty at all.

I grabbed the trolley, and slowly – only because I was worried that the spindly wheels were about to collapse under the weight of the load – crossed the quiet street back to Val's hideout. Everyone *must* have heard that. Her net curtains were up again and dropped as I approached the side gate. I strolled nonchalantly down the walkway at the side of the house, wobbly trolley in tow. Sanctuary.

I could feel the heady effects of adrenalin still pumping through me as I nodded to Val. She had joined me out back in her own wobbly, rickety way. As I emptied the trolley onto the broken paving, I felt alive, heroic. I expected a 'Well done'. 'Right, next load!' she said. My heart sank. But, as D.W. Winnicott wrote, 'We are poor indeed if we are only sane.'

'Did you see someone coming?' I asked, hopeful that she had.

She just stared at me. There was no sound and everything seemed to go still. Then she turned and walked inside, shaking her head. Three or four trolley loads of anxiety and sand later, the job was done. Although I could only remotely realise it at the time, this operation would provide not only a footing for the pond but for our relationship. I had assumed that *I* would establish this foundation, not Val. Yet everything she needed to learn about me was to be discovered in how I bedded in her precious pond the next spring. Meanwhile, I was off to New Zealand that very night, and didn't really expect to see her again. Or perhaps it was more a hope.

THE WAY OF TEA
February 1994

On arriving back in England from the relative simplicity of New Zealand, I went to a committee meeting where I was told that my position as Director of Training and Development was no longer required. I was to do everything I had been doing, but my title was forfeited. No satisfactory reasons were given, and after the meeting I drove over to Val's house under a dead grey sky. I felt wronged and unappreciated in the meeting; I felt sad and bitter in the car; I felt all of this, sitting on the sofa beside the pile of magazines. The barricade was somewhat diminished. So was I. But no matter what I was going through, at least I was not seventy-four and dying of cancer. Nature is all about proportion – my worries and concerns were finding their proper perspective when I saw them in relation to Val, her cancer and her isolation.

I waited for the 'Tea?!' and got up to follow Val into the kitchen. We had the rituals of the previous three months to get us back into where we had left off. Once in the kitchen, on this and other visits, we would safely discuss the garden while her kettle simmered and boiled on the back burner. It was an organic pattern become ritual, a genuflection towards

the altar prior to entering the chapel proper, a quiet invoca-
tion of the Gods. Almost every 'chat' in that kitchen was
about the garden, the garden which represented anything
from a mislaid future – 'It's no use putting in bulbs this year,
since I won't be here to see them, will I?' – to a symbiotic
relationship that would draw Val inexorably on – 'In summer
I'll have to get you to put up the bean poles for me. Tom
always did it and I wouldn't trust that man who does the
lawns to do it properly.'

My function in The Way of Tea, as practised ritualistically
in Val's kitchen, was to get the milk from the fridge and put
it back after Val had flooded my cup; salvage my tea bag and
bin it; and take the biscuits from the kitchen to the low table
that cowered in front of the overbearing sofa. I used to be
an altar boy, up early to ride my bicycle to church for the
six o'clock mass, waiting while the priest tested and re-tested
the red wine to make sure it was 'alright'. Val's was a more
simple ceremony with unembellished ordinary utensils, everything pared down to the essentials.

'Tea is nought but this,' said the Grand Tea Master, Rikyu,
'first you heat the water, then you make the tea. Then you
drink it properly. This is all you need to know.'

It was a matter of pride for Val that she should make the
tea in her own home, no matter how she felt. And I knew
not to interfere.

Gradually everything was being taken away from her. It
was the loss of the seemingly trite and insignificant – doing
her own shopping, wearing her own clothes, doing her own
ironing – that made it all so unavoidably clear: any control

she had over her life, or thought she had, was a delusion.
Nothing was so small that it would be overlooked in the
thorough, total, absolute termination of Val.

Returning from the kitchen, Val would begin to talk.
Sometimes the stories would be the same, sometimes different;
sometimes the same story told differently as she discovered
new meanings and new significances in things she had found
irrelevant or incomprehensible, up until now. I was the witness,
the one bequeathed her history; it was all coming to me. It
could leave me mesmerised, churned up, laughing, bleak. Or
bored out of my mind, as I stifled yawns, as I listened for the
umpteenth time to the same story. But then there would be
a new word, or a changed word, or the same word with a
different tone, all of which could signal a swing into a new
avenue of connection and emotion and recollection. And
suddenly, *there*, all that had been said before was heard within
a broader context. Everything changed, making what I had
thought insignificant, now central and essential and what Val
had only now discovered in herself, in her life, in her dying.
After fifteen minutes or an hour or two, she would stop
talking and look out at the yard, then at me, with a raise of
an eyebrow and a tired cheeky smile.

Outside I would rake the few leaves now half absorbed
into the ground and sweep paths and generally muck about,
looking busy, trying to feel I was doing something important.
Every once in a while, I would stop and stare, peering beyond
my anxiously stooped image reflected in the sliding glass doors,
to scan the lounge for a living being. And each time I did so
my chest would tighten, just a little, just in case. For why I

did not know until one day I looked in and saw Val writhing on the sofa, clutching her chest. I rushed inside, muddy-shoed and frowning. I knew what pill to get and where to pop it, and put it under her tongue. When we had first met I had worked out all her medication, which was legion. I was surprisingly methodical and calm, and her angina attack subsided remarkably quickly.

'I thought that was IT!' Val gasped.

'So did I,' I thought, and said it. Suddenly I felt really upset, but didn't show it. Practice makes perfect.

The peacefulness I had felt during the attack struck me as something new, something of myself I had not experienced so clearly before. In the time it took for me to walk back to close the doors to the garden and return to sit quietly beside her, beside the magazines, I had changed. I'd moved more into myself. I did not know, and still do not know, whether I saved her life, or saved her from some agony, or if the attack was already over by the time I got to her. I do know that through being there with her, I had begun to change, to rediscover abandoned aspects of myself. And somehow I had been expecting this. I could feel it. Val leaned back, deep into the womb of the sofa, and stared up at the ceiling for what seemed an age. She was staring at the dirty rectangular clouds corralled by the cornicing. To die under that! Then out to the garden, the fallen rake, the broken paving.

There was a sense of a great, almost religious intimacy in the room while I sat with her. All her defences were blown, and also mine. There was just she and I sitting there, exposed. Nothing needed to be said or done, *wei-wu-wei* as the Chinese say, doing-not doing. I felt not only a shift in myself, but that there was now some sort of 'us', a Val and Paul, a bond in calamity that excluded others, put them outside the chalk circle. We'd been through a minor skirmish together, two casualties.

After a while she asked me to help her up, and said, 'You'd better get on with the garden.' Like Tom's and Val's life, like my life, the garden was a very structured affair, where everything had once been planned and under control. An assault on Nature, but Nature will endure.

CRACK
Spring 1994

'So, what's your charity called again?'
    'Hospice Home Support.'
    '*Hospice* Home Support?'
    'Yup.'
    'And you helped set it up?'
    'Yes, there were about a dozen of us. Doctors, two nurses, Anna and Irene, you know them, and a friend of mine called Linda Hall asked me if . . .'
    Val cut me off, 'And it's called *Hospice* Home Support?'
    I would have to think quickly, I could see her next question now. 'Well, yes.'
    'And what sort of people go to a *ho*spice?'
    Think, think. 'How do you mean?'
    'You know what I mean.'
    '—'
    'I mean, isn't a hospice for people who are *dy*ing?'
    Yes it is, you know it is, and you're dying, and you know you're dying . . . 'People die in hospices, yes. But many people go to hospices for respite, or to give their family a break, or because they need a break from their fam . . .'
    'They're dying. Do you think I'm dying?'

God save us. 'Hospice means to cloak, Val, like to wrap in a protective cloak. That's why we use the word in the name of the charity. It's not like everyone we visit is going to die.'

'Do you think I'm going to die?'

'I don't know any more than you do, Val. Are you going to die?'

'Is that why you've come?'

'I don't know, Val. Something pulled me towards doing this. I don't know what exactly it was. I agree, it's a strange thing for a man my age to be doing. Maybe it's because I've been around a bit of death in my life. Perhaps that's got something to do with it. I expect I'll find out as I go along.'

She looked out to the garden, and said, 'You'd better get on with the pond.'

I walked out to the garden steaming. Her questions were fair enough, but she was taking no prisoners. It was a relief to be outside to clear my head. Gently I dropped the pond into the bedding of stolen sand and sat on the earth to carefully lower one foot into it, then the other, and pat the base gently down. *Festina Lente*, I wrote above each week of my diary, Proceed Slowly. Once I was sure the pond was well founded, I stood up gingerly. This tentative upward movement was accompanied by a sudden shot of adrenalin to the heart, as the cold air resounded with a pistol shot, *crack!*

'Oh no, oh God, no!' My left boot had split the bottom of the damn thing. I slumped down on the damp earth where only seconds before I had not been the sort of person who broke the ponds of old women dying of cancer.

'Fuckit fuck FUCKIT!'

Through the sliding doors I could see Val's face changing shades of blue in front of the television. She obviously hadn't heard a thing. I knew I could get some resin and fibreglass matting during the week, and quietly repair the damage during my next visit without Val knowing. She was not venturing out much, and even if she did I could get away with it if I just tossed some dirt in the bottom to cover the crack. She could no longer bend down to have a good look. As I saw it, there was no need to tell her anything: 'What you don't know can't hurt you' was the pearl of treacherous common wisdom that sprang too easily to mind.

I walked to the rear corner of the house and, in full view of Val, dragged the green hose down to the pond. I washed the pond out thoroughly and went and told Val what had happened, and what I planned to do about it. She listened, looked alarmed at first, but calmed down as I spoke. I repaired the crack the next visit, and she made the effort to come out and check what I had done. She was pleased, much more than I thought she would be, and this surprised me. Over the weeks that followed, the magazine pile between us on the sofa began to dwindle, slowly slowly dwindle. Sometimes it would go down by a couple of inches, sometimes by just one very thin magazine, but always it diminished. 'You can have truth without love,' the psychotherapist and author Anthony Lunt said to me many years later, 'but you can not have love without truth.'

There was not a day I arrived at Val's home, or later the hospital, or later still the hospice, that I knew what I would find or what would happen once I found it. There was not

a day that I left her without a myriad of experiences to assimilate, and a niggling doubt as to whether I would see her alive
again. I left also with a growing gratitude for accumulating
cumulus clouds, a beloved book, the smell of children's hair
and the sound of friends laughing, for Barolo and 1957
Corvette Stingrays and rain sheeting down, and the way
when, on foot, I would always take a different route back
from the one I took to get there.

THE JOHNNY FOREIGNER QUESTION
Spring 1994

Val could be a total pain in the arse, and so could I. It can be to a person's credit that others find them discomforting and challenging to be around, but Val could be just downright hostile. Even when feeling quite well, she could be superior, dismissive, and opinionated to the point of bigotry. Having nudged beyond the prognostic date for her funeral – 'outside the envelope' as it were – one day Val confronted me with a diatribe on 'foreigners'.

These 'foreigners', Val reliably informed me, the tabloid newspaper still warm on her knees, were 'flooding into Britain' and 'taking all the jobs'. She had plenty to say about it, 'let me tell you!'

And there sat I, Johnny Foreigner, having annexed part of her sofa for my own selfish purposes (somewhat accurate I'm afraid). I listened for a while; after all, Val was dying, I was a guest in her home, what could I say? I was still a little raw from the last committee meeting; I hadn't quite managed to leave it all outside the door.

'I'm from another country,' I said. 'I wasn't born here. So whose job do you think I'm taking?'

Val's mouth was open and ready to say something, and her

eyebrows were trying to meet in the middle of her forehead as she frowned. Her face said, 'That wasn't called for!' and I think, had she said it, she would have been right. I had closed another door on her, and from then on she either put aside those opinions or saved them for someone else.

At the same time Val told me more than once she was grateful I did not treat her as if she were dying – as partially deaf, disabled, incapable, a charity case, always right, et cetera – or, worse still, as though she were already dead – totally deaf, unable in every respect, utterly passive and so on. I believe a person who is dying easily becomes something other than a 'living' person in the eyes of those who assess themselves as 'living' purely on the basis that they have not yet grasped the fact that they too are heading towards death and may indeed get there before the 'dying'.

On that day the foreigner mowed the lawn, and afterwards Val trundled out to survey it in the way my dad would have done. She nodded her head and padded back to the kitchen, where she conjured a ten pound note out of her purse with a flourish and handed it to me. Johnny Foreigner Rips Off Dying Widow.

I had not expected this and was more than a little thrown as the note fluttered out of her purse to be waved unceremoniously under my nose. I was, after all, a volunteer, a volunteer administering my charity at her. But I knew to take the money, and Val's relief was clear.

'The last time I tried to give someone money for a little job they'd done for me,' she said, 'they told me they couldn't take it!' Drawing the tips of her thumb and forefinger close together, she added vehemently, 'I felt *that* small.'

'Ah,' I sagely replied, having felt I should accept the money without really knowing why. There seemed to be some part of me I could listen to, maybe even rely on, and it was not my head. Armed with Val's relief, I then had to think how I could explain the money to the charity.

'Well, the money will go to the charity,' I heard myself say. 'The one I helped set up,' I added; just to let her know something else about foreigners. 'It will be used to train more volunteers like me. So thank you very much, you're helping someone else who may want a visitor.'

She nodded, satisfied; she seemed a little more substantial. I followed her small, broad, floral-dressed frame to the sofa, where she sat quietly for a minute or two. 'People treat you like you're of no use to anybody anymore,' she said to her palms. 'Like they're afraid of you.' She stared down at her old hands as if she wondered whether she would have any use for them again. I had to admit, I was a little afraid of her.

My grandfather, Pop, came to mind. He had lived through the birth of the communist states, and the Great War, the war to end all wars, in which he was a prisoner of war in a German camp. He had dug tunnels. Then the Great Depression. He used to spend mornings digging holes along the side of the road for the government, then the afternoons filling them in. Pop liked digging holes. One day he and Nan, my mother's mother, had to get rid of an old refrigerator. Pop just went out the back and dug a hole big enough, and dumped the fridge right into it. It was the beginning of something. From that day on, nothing was thrown away. It was all buried out back.

After the Great War and the Depression, he lived through the Second World War, and the '100 Suns' of Hiroshima and Nagasaki. Pop kept living, right through Korea and Vietnam. He lived in a century where, as R.D. Laing pointed out, we killed about 150 million of each other – and put them in holes too.

Six years after my father's death, Pop had stayed in our family home and slept in what had been my parents' bed, not emerging from the room at all during the day. I knew he was ill, but that was all. I was disturbed one afternoon when my mother extracted me from the languid opiate reverie of the television, to tell me Pop wanted 'a word'. What *word*? I was in the computer business by then, making piles of money; I thought I was It. I hadn't talked with him in the twenty-three years I had been in his life. So why now? I went timidly into 'his' room, unexpectedly dark and cool on that humid day, feeling bewildered and anxious.

I stood by the low dark double bed in the gloom, heavy curtains shutting out all light as if it might kill him. Half under the heavy bedspread lay Pop. His mouth was working like a goldfish, big O shapes one after the other as if he was trying to breathe water. He seemed desperate to tell me something, but nothing was coming out of his mouth except a terrible wheeze. Out of the dim light there suddenly appeared the shocking spectre of his knarled blue-veined hand extending in my direction as he rose impossibly out of the sheet. I was hopelessly unprepared for facing death, even though I had seen so much of it on TV. Even though I had seen my father die. I was suddenly terrified and alone, I had no circuitry for this except fight or flight. I still wonder what it was he needed to tell me. I never saw my grandfather alive again.

HOW TO KNOW YOU'RE BORN
May 1994

Val and I sank back into the sofa, inhaling the sweet fragrance of freshly cut grass. Life was good. Dying was OK. A light breeze wafted in through the sliding doors, full of the promise of summer. She asked me to tell her about the hospice work, and so I told her a little about the training, how I had come to be involved with it, and then a question of my own, that I hadn't realised was there, came up: 'Val, I was wondering if it would be OK with you if I were to tell people about you, and what you're going through,' I said.

'Me! Tell people about me? Well, I never,' she said, pulling over and spluttering to a stop. She reached gingerly for her tea, her hand chubby from steroids, blue-veined and gnarled, a wedding finger spanned twice by gold.

'Yes, tell people about you,' I said. She sat still at this inter-section for a while, behind the wheel, the traffic of her mind diverted.

'Well, if you think it could be of some help, then you can tell as many people as you like.' She gave me one of those wide-eyed looks, as if I was crazy. 'But I can't imagine what you'd have to tell them . . .' she said as she turned towards me, ready for a little more fuel.

'Your story, Val, what you experience as you go along, and what it's like to be with you. It'd be much better than a whole bunch of theories. People can't relate to that stuff so well. It could be helpful. It could make a difference to someone, like how they could be with someone close to them who is very ill, or even how they live their own lives. I don't know, but that sort of thing. What do you think?'

'If you think it would help people, but I'm not sure you're thinking straight,' she said, looking at me askance, before she turned back to the garden, always back to the garden. She shook her head. I could see she was chuffed. It felt good she was pleased she could contribute something.

'Well, I never. I never would have thought it,' she said to herself.

After a while, and as was her habit, Val turned around to peer out of her net curtains. She hit pay-dirt: some schoolboys idling away class-time as they sat on her low brick wall.

'Look at them!' she grumbled. 'Skipping school, wasting their lives.' Was this the sort of thing I was going to tell people? There was a bitterness in her voice I was coming to recognise. It made me slow my movements as my heartbeat quickened – that little jolt of adrenalin. It made me go quiet as if dad had just pulled into the driveway.

'They don't know they're born! What a waste. What a *waste*!' she muttered, shaking her head as she turned back to the ending of her life. 'Why couldn't it have been one of *them* instead of me?'

I was shocked. I shouldn't have been, but I was. I had not heard anything like that from her before. Well, actually, I had.

But this was in a different league. I was shocked because I
hadn't really thought about it. And there was Val, seventy-
five years of age, and these kids were no more than twelve
or thirteen.

She hadn't finished. 'I've got so much more to live for. It's
not fair. It's just not fair at all. Young people these days; they
just waste their lives. They haven't been through a war or a
depression or anything remotely like it. They just take everything for granted. When I think of all the good men and
women who gave up everything, their lives and *every*thing,
so these kids could sit all day on my wall. And people don't
even bother to go out and vote. Makes you wonder what it
was all for. People come into this country . . .' she petered
out a bit there, but not for long.

'I really enjoy my life. I have my garden . . .' she paused.
Yes, the garden. 'And my friends . . .' she faltered. She had
begun to discover something unnamed in these anguished
hateful moments, something that she had been protecting
herself from for most of her life, something that lay in the
deep background of her being like a menacing theme tune
that played on quiet but distinct, reverberating to every beat
of her existence.

Val tried to go on. 'I look forward to things . . .' she searched
for her 'why' . . . 'To having another day . . .' Her voice had
become low and quiet, and I saw in her eyes confusion and
despair, as she struggled for that oxygen of the spiritual life:
meaning. It was sad to watch as she searched dejectedly for
the reason she should be saved, why she should be chosen,
given a place on the lifeboat, with us. It became deathly quiet

and still as we went down in the low little room. And I was listening, but little cogs turned inside me, small mechanicals operating on the same questions Val was faced with.

'Sometimes I accept it,' she said quietly, guiltily. 'Sometimes I'm quite angry about it. I imagine people think I've had my innings and that I shouldn't feel too bothered. But I do. I really feel bothered sometimes. I'm not dead yet, but people treat me like I am.' She looked up and caught my eye, and I saw tears welling in hers. 'Do you understand?'

From the other end of the sofa, from the other side of darkness, I said, 'I believe I do, Val, as much as I can from over here.'

She nodded and sat quietly for some time. 'You're the only person I can have a really good talk to,' she said with a sad smile and a raise of her eyebrows. We held each other's gaze for that extra moment. And I wondered as I looked into those long-lived watery eyes: was I living, or was I just pretending, a menace to my own destiny?

We sat there for a few minutes, looking into the garden until something inside Val seemed to say: 'To hell with all that!' and she steamed off purposefully towards teabags and milk, routed yet brimming with purpose.

BUM

The reddening nurse swung around as fiercely as she could while holding two heavy medical cases, and tried to face down Mrs Val Hall at the door.

As if to prove she was not an itinerant corpse, Val drew innocents into conflict. With no desire for resolution, she picked fights wherever and whenever she could. She had never suffered fools gladly, but now this preoccupation had taken on a whole new meaning, it had become her manifesto for re-election into the echelons of the living. She was an agent in her own life, able to stir things up a bit. The committee would have got rid of her by now.

There were grievances everywhere she looked, and she looked everywhere. On this Thursday, as I walked up her small driveway, the nurse was leaving. She was probably on her way to visit another patient suffering from God knows what in God knows what circumstances, and not expecting Val's parting volley.

'My!' Val had said, as if she had some most interesting, most delightful discovery to impart, 'You *have* got a very large bottom, haven't you!' Eyebrows at attention, chin out, Val beamed up at the nurse, who had wheeled around to face her. I stood there transfixed, delighted and appalled, while Val, full sail against the wind, blasted broadsides at the rest of the world.

The nurse just stood there, hands holding heavy bags, shoulders tense and burdened, looking down at Val's beaming face. A few seconds passed. They stood there, staring at each other. Val was very rude; but Val was very dying. Perhaps the nurse hoped for an apology, as her shoulders sank a little. But in the end she stood there, routed.

Having seen as clearly as I the collapse in the nurse's resolve, Val went on with the same tone of joyous discovery, 'Oh! Here's my hospice visitor. Do you know Paul?' She didn't. She left, no doubt to discover and rediscover, once safely ensconced in her car, the parting shots that would have blown holes in Mrs Val Hall.

It was not so much that Val was declaring war; it was more a testimony to her ability to wage one, should she choose. All she was saying, really, was, 'I am alive! Don't forget that. I can affect you. You can't ignore me yet. You can't pretend I'm not here. I won't let you!' It did not bother her one iota whether the person warranted this treatment or not; it was something that Val needed to do. I tried not to prune or sober Val (any more), not even when she had her sights set on me, and demonstrated a frontier willingness to pull the trigger. Since 'living' people are as a rule intimidated by 'dying' people, Val knew she could pretty much get away with anything she wanted to. Yet in truth it was not that these people were telling her she wasn't alive; it was Val wondering if she had ever *lived*. She found the possibility that she had not disturbing and potentially irrevocable. We padded inside, and I wondered if I would be next.

A PUZZLE

The visits flowed one into the next. They were separated by time but still we dipped our hats into the same stream. Val was being presented with 'puzzles', most of which would not and could not be answered in her lifetime. Instead, they required us both to reach deeper than the level they arose from; not to find an answer at all, but to make a change in position.

Val took pride in 'putting a brave face on it'. But this evasion only served to confirm the horror of the 'it' she felt the need to be brave in the face of. She was having radiation treatment at the time, and did not want to know how worried she was about it. Instead she thought, 'I'm having treatment so I must be getting better'. Her position no longer matched up with the gradual but obvious deterioration in her health, a deterioration that at times she seemed completely unaware of as she looked towards the results of her latest treatment. Because she was not anchored in reality, but in coping, she experienced massive mood swings and the understandable desire to, in Sigmund Freud's words, 'flee into health'. No matter my own secret hopes that Val might ask me for advice I also knew she could only be found where she was, and that is where I tried to be.

One day, while I was sitting in front of another lactose-laden cup of tea, Val said: 'I've been thinking about the end of it, Paul, how I could learn more about what might happen to me.' She was sitting facing towards me, spectacles folded and hanging down on a coloured cord across her chest, white hair brushed back off her open face – Einstein, looking at me with old watery eyes full of dreadful realisation. 'Couldn't bear to think of being in a lot of pain, you see,' she said. 'It's one thing I really don't want to have to go through. That and losing my marbles. I don't know which would be worse.' Neither did I.

I was twisted to my left to face her. It was a position I sometimes had to maintain for hours on that sofa, sitting there dirty and uncomfortable after a smoggy spring ride down the motorways on my Harley. Depending on how long Val wanted to 'chat', this could be another day I left with a crick in my neck. It made listening hard sometimes, and I should have said something.

But I'd been brought up a Catholic. So somewhere inside, in a little cubicle behind a black curtain, I believed I had to suffer, if I wanted to do anything worthwhile. Like be loved, or get to Heaven.

'So how do I find out about it?' she said.

'Have you thought of getting a couple of books, Val? Maybe something about someone who was seriously ill.' I didn't say 'dying' because I never knew whether this was a minute in which she was getting better, or a minute in which she would soon be dead.

'Read a book about *dy*ing?' Val was appalled. But curiosity

got the better of her, and she said, 'Are there *books* about it
– what's happened to people, I mean?'

'Yes, of course.' I said.

'Books about dying! It would be odd to read one, wouldn't
it?' she said. 'Have you?'

'A few,' I said. They hadn't helped me learn anything, of
course, nothing useful, but then I apparently wasn't '*dy*ing'.

'Oh, goodness. Why would you want to read something
like that?' she asked herself. 'I suppose it's something you
must be interested in. You must think it important, I suppose,'
she answered her own question correctly. 'Do you think it
would be a good idea for me to read one?'

'Well . . .' I was thinking. 'Have you ever been to France?'
I said, immediately realising that any other country would
have been a better choice.

'What on earth has *France* got to do with anything?' she
said, eyebrows raised, mouth agape, staring at her idiot Paul.

'Have you ever been to France, Val?'

She stared at me, then said, 'Yes, you know that already,'
but it didn't stop her telling me again. 'Only once, thank God.
Tom and I went and I can tell you we did *not* like it very
much. All of them acted like they couldn't speak English!
Would you be*lieve* it? And of course we didn't speak French,
why would we? So we just didn't get on with them. We didn't
go abroad together again after that. Although Tom kept going
off to Poland, of course, to see his woman.'

His woman. Oh, how I wanted to divert her onto this
track, toggle the right levers in the control tower. France was
fast proving to be a bad example, but having no alternative

I kept going. 'Well most people, if they knew they were going to France, would probably look at a map or read a guide-book or something about how to get there before they went, what other people knew about it, what sort of things go on there, that sort of thing. They wouldn't just set off, they'd want to know the . . . the possibilities.'

With an appreciative glance and a nod of her head, Val said, 'I'd like to read a book about dying.' But as far as I know, and I know only what she told me, she never did.

'And that reminds me,' she continued, not missing a beat, 'there's something else we need to talk about: home or hospice. That's the puzzle for today, and you can think about it while you do the pond.'

Val's vision of the pond became more ambitious with each small success. And as long as your project is not finished, you can't die. So there was always more to do on the pond. I sat down with her an hour or so later, leaving my muddy shoes at the door, and asked how far she had got in her thinking about this particular puzzle.

'Everyone knows if you go into a hospice there's only one way you're ever going to come out again, and that's in a box. So I'm not going in,' she said. She was clear about most things. I'd been clear about most things too, before I'd met Val.

'Has someone suggested you should go into the hospice?'

'Irene and Anna think it would be a good idea, so I can get some proper rest. They should know I suppose, being nurses. But they said I might even *like* it in there. I can't imagine that could be true, so I'm not going. What do you think?'

'You wouldn't enjoy being taken care of for a while, Val?'

'They need the beds for very ill people,' she said dismissively. 'Not someone like me. I'd feel rotten if they gave me a bed that someone else really needed, so that's that. Do you think I should go?'

'Did Irene or Anna say the hospice was short of beds?'

'No, they said it was quiet at the moment. Which I suppose means business is down. Maybe that's why they want to get me in there, to be done with me while there's no rush on,' she laughed, but it was hollow. 'I just don't know if it's the right thing to do or not. It's a puzzle.'

'If you don't like it you can tell them to take you home again, Val, or I could always come and get you.'

'Yes, but would you visit me if I was in there? I know it's a long way out of your way, and you're very busy with everything.'

'Of course, Val, of course. I'll follow you around wherever you end up.' Well perhaps not *wherever*. Not yet anyway.

'There are stories that they put things in the food so that people don't last very long in there, if you know what I mean,' she said, opening her eyes wide. 'We'll just have to see about it when the time comes, won't we?' she said, turning towards me sternly. 'So it's no use you lot trying to talk me into it, because I'm quite capable of making up my own mind, thank you Very Much!'

And so the conversation went on for another hour or so, around and around the same ground, Val with no Gods or dreams to lean into for warning, guidance, or support; her hardback illustrated copy of Omar Khyyam's *Rubaiyat* her single spiritual solace, a precious gift from Tom during the early days of their relationship. She used to skim through it occasionally, more and more as the myeloma progressed. It did her pretty well for religion and psychology and meta-physics, which may have been very wise.

'I never met her,' she said out of the blue, and looked down into her hands for some suggestion as to whether she should carry on. I said nothing.

After a minute she carried on, 'I gave him an ultimatum. A direct order really. He said he loved her. He said he wanted to live with her; over there or over here, it didn't matter to him. He just wanted to be with her. Said she made him happy.' Val looked forlorn and exhausted. She stared down into the carpet, unable to meet my eyes.

'But I was his wife, and that's what he had to understand,' she said as she shook her head, seeming to wonder if she wanted to hear any more of her own story. She leaned forward, forearms on her thighs, her right hand worrying the two bands on her wedding finger, marriage and eternity.

'He had to go over there every so often, it was part of his work,' she said, needing to talk and at the same time humil-iated by what she was saying. She glanced at me, and my face would not have shown how sad I felt. 'He met her somehow and that was that, apparently. He said he loved her, and that she loved him. But I told him I was his wife and I wasn't ever going to give him a divorce. No matter what.' She was telling me what had happened, but also showing me something of what it was to be her in life. She had been left by her mother; adopted only to be replaced by unexpected siblings; and then to be married and threatened with being left and replaced again. She would be having none of it.

'We argued about her for months, but I wasn't going to budge. And Tom knew it. I wish he'd just kept quiet about her; I didn't have to know. We hadn't had sex for so long, what difference did he think it was going to make to me if he loved someone else. In the beginning I told him it was none of my business if he wanted to see her. But he wasn't going to leave me for some woman in Poland. He wasn't ever going to leave me. No matter what.' But he did. Like my father. Val just sat there for a while, leaning forward over her hands in supplication.

'In the end I told him he wasn't to see her again. Not ever.' Val leaned back into the sofa and sat in silence for a minute.

'Things were never right between us from then on. He saw her once more after that, I'm sure of it. But I pretended I didn't know. They wrote to each other for a while. I know that because I used to get the mail.'

She sat perfectly still for a while, then said in a low voice, 'I'm not sure I did the right thing now. I don't think he ever really got over her. But he stayed with me.' She turned towards me. 'He always tried to do what was right,' she said, then stared back out towards the garden. 'Things weren't the same between us again, and we never talked about her after that. For all I know she might still be alive and not know Tom's dead. It's a strange thought, that. She might still love Tom, and not know he's not around to be loved anymore . . . But he was my husband, and she'd no right to make him love her.'

To make him love her. Val didn't think anyone could ever love her, I saw that then, hidden in those words. And they triggered something similar in myself.

It was a long visit that day. Val's mind swung from memory to memory, like a weathervane in a gathering storm. And later on, when I was gently chuckling away at some dark humour that had blown in, she suddenly turned to me and by a look in her eyes fixed me dead. 'If I begin to lose my dignity,' she said, 'will you help me to take my life?'

Part Two

Is Now, And Ever Shall Be

SAMANTHA

1977

Samantha died brutally on the morning of my psychology examinations. Her death different from my father's death at enrolment, in that this time I made it through breakfast. But again death came unannounced, and again I was picked up like a dead leaf and blown to dust. I had got ready to leave for the campus, and wanted to say goodbye to Samantha before I left. She was nowhere to be found, and I'd become more and more unsettled by each quiet forgetful room.

I looked and called for her through the house and in the back garden. I looked out the front of the house, and all I found was traffic banking up outside the gate. But where was Sam?

There was the unusual sight of people gathered on the road itself, all appearing bewildered and lost.

Maybe I had somehow missed her inside. The people were just standing there, still and quiet, staring at something lying on the road, quiet and still.

I called her, 'Samantha. SaMANtha!' I couldn't explain it, but I felt myself beginning to panic, really panic.

Some of the people on the road had begun to stare over at me. I stared back at them. I felt like I was being sucked

into something, some black hole, some infinite gravity. One
of them began a faltering approach.

An inner tide drew me back inside, to have another look
for Samantha. From room to vacant room, more desperate
with each one, then out once more to the back yard, out of
breath from tension, out, out.

As I called her name again and again, I recognised a strange
resistance to returning to the front of the house, to the scene
on the road. Instead, I returned to my bedroom. Without a
thought I fetched my beloved cotton raincoat, long and sand-
coloured. I wore it everywhere, even in summer.

Samantha's things were left all over the floor of our room.
Somehow these things were more than left, they were abandoned. Going out the front door, beginning to switch off
inside I made for the midst of the people on the road. That
same front door; the porch; dad. I could not, could not, just
could not bear it.

The people on the road seemed bewildered. Sam was
unmoving and silent on the road. Her tongue lolled grotesquely
out of her open mouth, and down to the tarmac. Blood had
already dried on her lips.

'Sam.'

Nothing. Her nickname was Sam-I-Am. That's what I called
her. She'd answer to that.

Quieter, more softly, closer to her ear, 'Sam-I-Am'. My
voice went then, cracked and shook. But I held it all in, forced
it to stay down.

Nothing.

Her body. My coat. The people standing around. I became

alone in the midst of their shadows, moving amongst them in my own inner disintegrating world. I lay my coat on the road beside the limp inanimate body, and rolled Sam over and onto it. A pair of hands made to help me without actually coming into contact with the corpse, hovering as if bestowing some arcane blessing. I swaddled Sam, nice and snug on this warm morning. I was numb and cold. I could see only *her* body in *my* coat. I could find only nothingness between myself and the people talking at me on the road, as though I were five fathoms down, and aware of mumblings and movement far above on the surface.

I held Samantha devotedly in my arms, devoutly. She was surprisingly heavy. I walked past the familiar houses of my youth, the neatly trimmed lawns, the brilliant flourishing trees. I wasn't connected to this green young world any more. I made my way in a one-man funerary procession to the vet's half a mile away.

Once in the waiting room, I found myself quickly ushered out between the rows of lowered eyes, carrying this most embarrassing, most shameful and unwanted patient. We moved along the alley at the side of the brick building, down to the basement where the nurse opened a wooden door and snapped on the light. I saw a room well stocked with full rubbish sacks and felt suddenly disorientated. Why on earth had she directed us down here?

The nurse said nothing, just stared fixedly into the basement room, her head twisted grotesquely away from me. 'She's *dead*,' I said. That was the first time I had said it, 'She's *dead*.' As the words came out I clicked on like the light bulb: of course, the rubbish sacks were the burial finery of once-beloved pets. These animals, the Souls who had been so keen, so necessary, they were rubbish now. There were other dogs here, in those terrible bags. Why are people like this? Why do they behave this way? I felt like a solitary ambassador of some unclassified species, sharing few of the common sensibilities that gathered the bulk of mankind together. I bore the Queen of Beasts, Sam-I-Am, my Golden Labrador.

I looked for a place I thought Sam would like to lie in. I circled like a dog, sensing the space. When it found us, I set her tenderly on the cool floor, still and snug in my trusty coat. I took that first step back, away, like at dad's funeral. I turned to leave, to be met by 'Your coat!' from the nurse. I glared at her with my best seventeen-year-old's I'd-kill-you-right-now-if-I-had-a-machine-gun sort of glare, and stomped out to the dismissing sound of the light being snapped off behind me. I left Sam alone, in the no-one-elseness of the dark. What a bastard. Something deep and essential within me – click! – gave up its attempt at life, some deep engine within ceased its constant hum and vibration. It would be years before even a hint of it would be found again.

I walked home, gathered my things, and tried not to notice the remains of Samantha's life strewn across my room. I walked out of the front door, over the cool quarry tiles. I crossed the road to the bus stop, and tried not to notice Samantha's blood on the asphalt. I thought only of a timely bus, so I could make it to the lesser examinations of that day.

I was not thinking of her, I was feeling her, dead and alone

in a dark hard world of the redundant and the replaceable.
Sam I am.

Forty minutes on the big yellow bus, and I made my way
up through a small wooded park to the university. I met a
girl I knew. I did what I could to tell her what had happened
not thirty feet from where my father had died. The bewildered girl said something to that young man about the crowds
of people around the campus. She went to touch my arm,
but pulled away at the last moment. Death catches. She turned
away from me, as I had. Then she walked off, without looking
back, leaving me alone, in the dark. Click!

THE END OF THE LINE
May 1994

'Will you help me to take my life?'

I'd had patients threaten to kill themselves before, but this was the first time one had asked me to help. It felt just the same. Nothing in life or in books or in lectures had prepared me for it. A quiet dread rose in my body, but I caught a piece of my mind, and it said, '*That* is a really difficult question.'

'That's a really difficult question, Val.'

She quietly nodded and returned her gaze to her hands in her lap. 'Well, sometimes when I'm feeling a bit low, which is more often than I want to, I wonder what's going to happen next.'

'Mmm,' I said, fruitlessly wondering what was going to happen next, spending way too much time out there, leagues away. Then back to Val and the room and feeling sad. I kept still. I waited.

'And the worst thing I think isn't that I'm going to die, because we're all going to do that, that's obvious. It's not *that* that really bothers me, it's that I might lose my dignity or lose my mind; not be able to think things through or make myself understood. Those are the things that frighten me most.'

She looked down at her specs, folded on her chest. She slowly opened them, and inspected them for dust. She put them on, and took them off again. She re-checked them for dust, folded them very deliberately, and rested them back on her chest. It was very important she did this.

'That's as long as the pain is under control of course, but Irene and Anna tell me that it's very rare these days for someone to suffer much pain. They say that's pretty much all under control, except for a poor few. I might be one of them I suppose, and I don't want that, I certainly don't want to have to face *that*, but that's not what's really bothering me.'

'It's that you could lose your dignity and maybe your mind,' I said.

'Mmm. That's the puzzle I'm trying to solve.'

'And what would that be, losing your dignity?' I felt upset. I wanted to know. I wanted her to see that if she told me I would know. But then, how could I?

There was a long pause as she fiddled with a piece of hard dead skin on the edge of a fingernail. 'I don't like people doing things for me,' she said. 'You're all right, because you wait until you're asked, but other people often don't do that. They come in, make the tea when I can do it, they want to do the housework when I can do it. They don't even ask sometimes, they just push in and take over. Well it's *my* home, and if they are going to be like that then I'd rather they just didn't come. I'm not an *in*valid.'

'But . . .'

'But, I *might* be. That's what I don't much like the thought of – people doing *every*thing for me and me being *use*less, no use to anybody. I couldn't bear just sitting there, dribbling down my front. Or something worse!' she wiped her palms along her dark blue trousers. 'I think that as long as I'm of some use, then life's worth living. Like, when you come here, I can see I'm teaching you things about dying, as well as it being the other way round.' She turned to look at me way over here and said, 'That's right, isn't it?'

'Yup, it is right, Val, yes.' Even though what I was teaching her, I couldn't imagine, even though I'd been so sure that was why I'd come.

'So with you it's not a problem. Yet,' she said with a sad smile and reddening eyes, 'and it better not become one!' I felt such warmth from her, wafting out towards me.

'Some people just haven't a *clue*, and then I have to just *sit* there, *smi*ling. If I lost my marbles what use would I be, to myself or anyone else for that matter? I wouldn't be able to solve any more of the puzzle of dying, would I? And don't think I haven't noticed you haven't answered my question.'

'Have *you* answered it? Would you end your life if things got too bad?'

'That's what I've been thinking about, and how to do it. I've got enough pills in the fridge to stop an elephant, and I think that's the way I'd do it. Just take the pills and go to sleep. For good,' she said, and paused in the relieving drowsiness.

'I don't think I could harm myself, if you know what I mean. I couldn't cut myself, or throw myself out the window or anything like that. I don't think I'd have the courage, and I can't imagine how anyone could do that. I've thought of crashing my car, but even then I don't think I could let myself drive into a wall or anything. And if I did I might end up hurting someone else and I wouldn't want that on my conscience. I've thought that even if I *could* harm myself, I might end up just being very badly injured and in a lot of pain. Then they might lock me up until I die.'

We sat with that for a while – being locked up until you die. It felt familiar. We're in our cells. There's nothing worthwhile we can find to do, so we just watch what everyone else does, and do that. Like them, we pretend it's all worth it, and we don't think about being in our cells. We try not to think about where we've ended up, when we'd expected so much. We try to forget what we wanted, we try hard to believe that what we've got is what we wanted, that what we've got is better. We try to forget who we are, which comes surprisingly easily.

So Val and I sat there, looking out at the garden, at the natural cycle of life, death and renewal that suffers the assaults of man.

'So what I'm left with, I've decided, is pills,' she said, with raised eyebrows that immediately fell into a frown. 'They would do it *to* me rather than me doing it, if you see what I mean. That part of the puzzle I've worked out. The puzzle now is this: what if I can't manage it by myself, what if things get so bad I just can't manage it, what then? That's the bit of the puzzle I can't solve. That's why I'm asking you, Paul, if you will do it *for* me if I can't?'

She stared across at me. I surfed for years before I learned to swim. And once I stood high on top of a waterfall, one step away from the Definite. Once I'd stood right on the edge of an underground platform, only one step away from a fall down to the tracks and the train barrelling towards me. I watched it coming, hurtling hot air and aluminium. Three memories, all in a split-second. Val stared at me.

'I can't give you a yes or a no, Val. I just can't know the answer to that now. It would be ignorant to answer. I'm not saying yes, and I'm not saying no; I'm saying that I can't know the answer to that from here, from where we are now.' Where was this stuff coming from? It sounded . . . OK.

Her gaze returned to her hands in her lap, and her frown dissolved from her brow. 'I thought you might say something like that,' she said. 'And I thought that would be good enough for me.' She leaned back into the chaos as her eyes wandered over the garden.

'If you'd have said yes, I would have wondered what you thought of me – perhaps you couldn't care less.' She smiled up at me. 'So I was hoping you wouldn't say yes, and you wouldn't say no. So we'll see, won't we?'

'We will, Val,' I said quietly. 'We will.'

And we did.

CHRISTINE

'I haven't heard a word from Christine,' Val would say as I followed her to the sofa. So many visits began this way. It was heart-breaking.

'I haven't heard a word from Christine.' Sometimes bitter, sometimes forlorn, sometimes mystified.

These were the repeated words of the summer months, as I sat smothered in Val's stuffy claustrophobic home. These words swirled in the air, along with the dust caught in the rays of Val's dying, settling on everything, almost invisible but taking the shine off it all.

'I haven't heard a word from Christine.' A pitiful look towards me as if I was keeping Christine from her. If I could get Val to say something, or do something, or see something, Christine would answer, would return to her dying mother, would be with her until the end. To the end.

'I haven't heard a word from Christine.' Week after week, month after month, these words re-established us in Val's world of the unmanageable. It was as if this one statement entirely defined her now: utterly powerless in the face of the insurmountable ending of her life. Christine had become the one most evocative and consequential puzzle. Other than that of how to remain alive, forever.

'I haven't heard a word from Christine.' Her daughter's life was some vague event happening in New York, something to do with computers. And somehow Val had come to believe that her daughter was in the hands of an iniquitous psychoanalyst. Val didn't much consider the possibility that she had been the cause of her own alienation from Christine. She laid the blame for the rent in the fabric of their relationship squarely on the shoulders of this shrink.

'I haven't heard a word from Christine.' Christine did not respond. Not to letters; not to telephone calls. And this went on for months. In the beginning Val tried to convince herself, through trying to convince me, that Christine must be busy with very important things (relative, that is, to a dying mother); that on her return from some vital national or international business assignment, she would hear of Val's plight and come at the gallop. It was obvious that, up until now, Val hadn't been very interested in her daughter's life.

'I haven't heard a word from Christine.' I felt sorry for Christine as well. In my experience of Val, and from what she had said of herself, I thought she might have been a severe mother. It was possible that the only viable and healthy response was for Christine to cut herself off from further exposure.

Equally I pitied Val her feebleness. Faced with the yawning gap in their relationship, Val was undone. The poignancy of what was left *un*said was utterly depressing, as she tried to fill the space in the relationship with assumptions. She poured fantasies into the chasm where a bond with her one child should have been. She did not appear to pause and wonder if she had loved her child; if her child was right to stay away; if Christine's need was greater than Val's.

She began to feel that I, too, would not want to see her. She cancelled my visit one week and called me the following weekend to say, 'You don't need to come this week, I'm still not feeling very well.' She sounded angry, but more than that, she sounded hurt.

'What sort of not well?' I said.

Silence.

'Physically or emotionally?'

'Both.' Curt, like a child with her bottom lip stuck out. I knew *that* place.

'So you don't want me to come then?' I'd watched people gently tease me out, so I had a feel for what to do.

'I'm not much fun to be around at the moment,' she said, 'I'm feeling a bit low.'

'You don't have to be fun to be around, Val. It's not like you have to entertain me or anything.' I knew this was right, but I wasn't sure it was true.

'Yes, but I'm sure you've got things you need to be getting on with.'

'How about I come,' I said, 'and if you don't feel like having me there, you can just tell me to shove off. How would that be?'

'Ha! Well, if you're sure it wouldn't be too much trouble.'

'I'll see you Thursday,' I said, which I did.

It was June – the cricket, the boiling traffic, the rains Wimbledon brings in. Val took me out to the rectangle of warm back garden allocated to vegetables and instructed me on the 'proper' installation of bean poles. She seemed to be making it up as she went along, an authority on bean pole setting, a master class. The poles were on a shelf in the garage, perched above Val's defunct and dust-covered car. The garage itself was a tomb for Tom's abandoned tools and machinery. It reminded me of my grandfather's garage: a sanctum bulging with the paraphernalia of mechanised man. All *useful* things, things not yet buried in the back lawn. His garage was the greasy altar at which, as a boy, I'd longed to be initiated, only to be left a pagan.

The bean pole day was a success (they did not fall down when the wind blew), and it was a welcome respite from talking about the letters, the phone calls, the letters, the phone calls. Each disappeared into the Bermuda Triangle that was Val's fantasy of her daughter's life. Perhaps not quite disappeared, as there was a faint echo in return, and it niggled at Val continuously. It was the deletion of messages from Christine's answer machine.

Val finally asked me about it, once she was clear she already knew, 'What are those beeps on Christine's phone?'

You know, Val, you know. 'When you leave a message?' I asked.

'Well I'm hardly *speak*ing to her, am I?' she snapped. She glared; she wanted a loaded gun.

'You said you'd stopped calling her, Val. That's all I meant.'

Beep.

'The beeps,' I said, knowing she knew I knew, 'mean messages have been left on her machine.'

'One for each message?' she asked, playing it out.

'Yup, usually.'

'So when I phone Christine to leave another message, and there aren't so many beeps or no beeps at all, what does that mean?' Sometimes Val would push me along in front of her, a shield against the assaults of reality.

'It means messages have been deleted, Val.'

'Ah,' she said bitterly. Palms slapped down upon floral knees, 'Tea!'

Christine did not come up again for a couple of weeks after that, which was in itself a significant appearance through non-appearance. Then Val showed me what she had been thinking over that time, 'Well, all I can say is, whoever Christine has got checking her messages while she's away is going to get A Piece Of My Mind. If I ever get hold of her!'

'Someone's checking her messages?' I said. I knew in my bones this wasn't it, some things people say go into me and just don't sit right. Val knew it too, but it had to be played out.

'Obviously!' she said. 'And whoever she is, she must be deleting them without even passing them on, the silly cow.' In Val's mind, the 'Silly Cow' had joined the 'psychoanalyst' to ruin Val's relationship with Christine. There was only one thing for it, so Val began to leave messages for the Silly Cow as well, telling her to stop deleting the messages and tell Christine that her mother was dying. It may seem crazy, but it showed just how fraught Val was. 'This world is a comedy to those who think', wrote Horace Walpole, 'a tragedy to those who feel.'

I listened to Val talk about 'her' and 'him' many times, in many versions, for many hours, and since she did not ask my view, I simply listened but, as I did, I found the situation more and more moving and more and more agonising.

She just could not get her head around the fact that her resiliently silent daughter could know Val was dying, and not be drawn out because of it. But it was becoming too obvious, surely. I was wrong about that. Val struck upon the desperate possibility, even *hope*, that her daughter was dead or ill, and so was just not able to answer.

This idea was asylum, respite from what Val saw as rejection by her only child. It meant that the love and forgiveness she wanted from Christine *would* have been given if only Christine *could* have given it; that everything could and would have been all right; that there was no problem between them that could not have been overlooked or forgiven. It could mean anything Val wanted it to mean, and at that point anything was preferable to how it was.

Val contacted 'The Authorities', with the aim of having them uncover her daughter's plight, thus projecting her own predicament all the way to New York. Val was very tense over these months, months during which she tried desperately to deny what she knew in the myelomic marrow of her bones: that Christine no more wanted to know the dying Val than she had wanted to know the living one; and that this lack of interest was based on how Val had treated her.

With the involvement of the police, Val dreaded the response she longed for. So when at last the news arrived that Christine was neither dead nor ill nor kidnapped nor missing, but mulishly alive and well in New York, Val's guilt-ridden hopes collapsed into a guilt-ridden despair. The news was at once a relief and a catastrophe. Where Val wanted reconciliation, she had found a vast and unbridgeable silence.

It was finally unavoidable, Christine wanted nothing to do with Val. It was a deep and bitter blow, not only to Val's vision of the relationship – that all was, is, and shall be well – but to her *version* of it – that it was Val who was the victim. It assaulted the narrative line she had wanted to impose upon her dying, that common plot of the beloved parent surrounded by the loving and bereft children, no matter how they had treated each other in the past.

The peculiar benefit of knowing this was an end to the anguish of not knowing, a resolution into a harsh clarity. Val had not been much of a mother. That was that. Nothing could be done about it now. It could not be put right. But nothing was firm in Val anymore, all was movement and change. It quickly became like her dying – sometimes she was, sometimes she wasn't. It depended.

She doggedly started sending postcards to Christine, hoping she would not be able to resist at least a glance. Her eyes would unavoidably fall on 'not long to go' or 'before the end', in large wobbly script. There was, defiantly, no response.

'I can't believe it,' Val said. 'I can't believe that a daughter would not bother to contact her Own Mother. Her own *Dying* Mother. It just doesn't seem possible, does it? I mean, I just can't fathom it, can you?'

Yikes! 'Well, yes, I can,' I said. 'That *is* what's happening.'

Christine had told the police that she wanted Val to leave her alone.

'Yes, no, but I mean you wouldn't do that to *your* mother, would you?' she said. She needed someone a bit nearer, someone within range. I could feel it.

Wouldn't I? 'I couldn't rule that out, Val,' I said. 'It would depend on how we got on.'

'No, but I mean you wouldn't do *that* would you? Not to Your Own Mother!' She was desperate for Christine to be wrong.

'That would depend on what sort of relationship I had with her, Val,' I said, not so comfortable either, at my end of the sofa. 'It isn't out of the question.'

'Well, what sort of a child would that make *you* then?'

'Adult', I thought, but I didn't say it. Maybe I should have.

'She's not giving me so much as a *chance*,' she said, furious, barely able to contain herself. 'For God's sake, I've told her how sorry I am and that I want her here. There isn't going to be another chance. I've told her she's made a big mistake, and it's going to stay with her for the rest of her life. She can be very stubborn. When I'm gone, she isn't going to be able to do *a thing* about it! I'm thinking of her as well as me.

'I haven't been a perfect mother, I can see that. But she should still be with me when I'm dying. I *am* the only mother she's ever going to have. It's this psychoanalyst that's put her up to it you know, I'm sure of it. She would never want to do anything like this to Her Own Mother. He must be keeping Christine away from me by telling her all sorts of stories about me. That's what they do, isn't it?'

Val had been reading something like this in the newspapers. They were saying that counsellors brainwashed their patients into believing their parents had sexually abused them. I had stopped reading the papers. They were too toxic. It was like getting up in the morning and drinking a quart of printer ink before going out onto the streets, poisoned and anxious.

One Thursday afternoon, with still no response from Christine, Val asked, 'What would you do about Christine if you were me?' It was a good question. I stared from the sofa out into the garden, our garden. I told Val I would think about it, and I could see by her nod she was pleased. We sat there softly, quieted, while the cancer ate away at her without rest, without reason and without remorse.

WEED
June 1994

June was weeding time, and for me it was a bit of a guessing game – weed or plant? Weed: *a herbaceous plant not valued for use or beauty, growing wild and rank, and regarded as cumbering the ground or hindering the growth of superior vegetation* – replace *herbaceous plant* with *Val* and you've pretty much got a hold of the western world's view of her. Weed or plant?

With her hands on her hips, as she stared down into a world even lower to the ground than her, she would demand, 'Where's my (unintelligible Latin words) gone?!' These inspections were few and far between, with her barely able to make the round trip from sofa to garden and back again. We live our lives in ever diminishing circles.

'You'd better come back inside before I've nothing left,' she'd say, and I'd down tools and follow her inside and inwards. I knew geraniums though, Val loved her geraniums. Crooked and old looking and bulging in odd places, they looked arthritic. But catch them at the right time, and they gave out the most vibrant flowers.

'They're going to give me chemo,' she beamed at me, fists clenched and raised as if she was going to beat her breast,

King Kong with Kancer. She'd obviously been saving this news up as a bit of a treat for me.

'Oh (No!)?'

'Well, you could be a little more enthusi*a*stic', she said. But I didn't feel enthusiastic, not a bit of it. I crumpled inside, like a caving in of some subterranean tunnel that Val and I had been digging with spoons, when we should have been sleeping in our prison bunks. I dreaded what was to come. But if I was Val, I would probably have done the same as her. 'Even though it be from bad to worse,' Washington Irvine wrote, 'it is often a comfort to shift one's position and be bruised in a new place.'

'Sorry, Val. So how did this come about?' I had to be completely out of her way now and let her steer us – it was the only way I could be *with* her.

'Well, the doctor came up with it out of the blue,' she said. 'I didn't think they'd give chemo to someone my age, but there you are. It just goes to show you, doesn't it?'

She glanced at me with her eyebrows raised, 'I thought they'd given up on me, but I start next week.'

Christ. I nodded and said, 'And side effects? How might the chemo affect you, did they happen to say?'

'Yes, they did!' she said and straightened on the sofa. 'They said that if I responded well to the treatment, it could knock the myeloma on the head. Isn't that wonderful!?'

I said, 'That's what they told you?'

'They told me I might feel a little ill at times, and I could lose a bit of hair.' She turned to beam at me, 'But that's not much of a price to pay for being well again, is it?'

'No, Val, it wouldn't be.' I was beginning to lose a bit of hair right then and there. And I didn't know what the doctors had said to her but Val was sure, and I could only find her where she was.

None of this stopped her from talking about dying. It had always been as if Val were twin sisters, incommunicado with each other. Like Christine and Val. One was being carried inextricably towards death, the other waited for her own inevitable and indisputable cure: one sentenced, the other reprieved.

The sisters had been there from the beginning. Almost in the same breath Val could ricochet from funeral arrangements to the harvest of spring beans and back again. At times I had no choice but to play the part of her alter ego. On her behalf I would have thoughts or feelings she could not face, such as the chemo. It was as if I had to experience, within the confines of myself, all that she disavowed and neglected, and it felt as if she had just sentenced me to a course of chemotherapy, a despairing course that would end in death.

Either the doctors had told her that the chemotherapy would cure her or they had not, it made little difference. Val would be cured. Val would die. And one of the side effects, not listed on the bottle, was that the intense pressure to make things up with Christine had gone.

Val sat there on the sofa, resolute, floral-dressed in hues of pastel pinks and blues. Her hands opened and closed in her lap, as if kneading the milk of eternal life from the breast of technology.

A BIT OF HAIR
July–August 1994

Each dose of chemo left Val half-dead at best, but she kept on keeping on. Steadfast and obstinate, she *would* be well. This warmed her. It sung in her.

It was the return home after each treatment that began to get to her, as much as the treatment itself. No husband or daughter, no one to say hello to or to reassure her. No one there when she woke up late at night, empty in the empty little house. No one there as she worried she was about to die. Is this It? Each return was worse than the last, which had been the worst so far. When I could, I would pick her up directly from hospital after the chemo. Or I would visit her in the hospice if she had got that far. Sometimes I would be waiting for her when she was dropped off at home. But more often than not she came back alone, and when she opened the door, the house was dead.

Up until now, Val had hated the idea of a cleaner. But her isolation was erosive. She surrendered another part of her life, the place of 'doing' for herself. I pitied whoever was to step into the breach, they were going to get a hard time from Val – they would be stealing her life, showing her how weak and pathetic she had become.

She would hate them for this.

Her hair reflected how fast she was losing her grip, and the paucity of life left. And then one day, from behind the watery glass, she emerged bedecked with a hairdo that could best be described as heroic. She beamed up at me, enchanted with her brand new head.

'So! What do you think?' was the first thing she said, patting the woolly diving bell on top of her head as we submerged into the sofa.

'It must make you feel more comfortable, Val.' She was upset at losing her hair. But it was such a small price to pay for being well. I was sad to see this happen to her. It was cruel and pointless and I knew.

'Oh, it does, it does. The lady who brought them was ever so nice.'

Them? Perhaps she'd rounded up a whole herd.

'She was *lovely*!' Pat, pat. Surely it would soon begin to purr. 'I spent ages trying different ones on, and finally decided on this. I didn't want anything too different from my real hair, and thought most people wouldn't even notice it wasn't my own. What do you think?'

The wig was bold and definite and could not be overlooked. 'It's very *you*,' I said. She was pleased, pat pat.

I thought of Val when I wasn't with her. I wondered how she felt waking in the morning as I woke to my day; I thought about her having to climb up onto the raised white plastic seat on her loo, as I sat secure and grounded; I thought about her washing her tired flagging body with a luke-warm flannel, as I stood robust under a steaming hot shower; I thought about her exhaustion from taking up to an hour just to dress herself, while I yanked on clothes in a couple of minutes. In my mind I was with her through the breakfast she would prepare and only stare at. I thought of her through the day that meant little more to her than that she had made it. She had won the fight for that day, to sit there, in front of the TV. And then at night, when she would be getting into bed not knowing if she would wake. These things would remain to an extent an unbridgeable gap in experience between us. If I had a headache I might feel a little sorry for myself, while if it was her, she would worry it was a brain tumour. She would think, 'This could be It.'

After chemotherapy Val would either talk me through the treatment, in detail, or she wouldn't say a thing about it. Either way, she was clear how much better she must *necessarily* be feeling. I was beginning to relax around her; I was beginning to relax around myself. And it was similar for her. She went from wearing the wig, to wearing the wig and talking about wearing it, to wearing the wig and talking about not wearing it. Then one day the sparsely haired pate of her twin brother floated up to the door wearing a pastel blue-floral dress.

I found it hard not to stare and felt more than a little stirred by the intimacy of the place I had found in her life. How totally exposing it all was. I'd become a companion no more contentious or threatening than her teapot. And she wasn't so scary. Scared, for sure. Like me.

Suddenly, we'd been talking about something else, when

the sleeping question reawakened, 'So, what would you do about Christine if you were me?'

'I've thought about that, Val,' I said, and she smiled and gave her shoulders a shrug of anticipation. She was a real box of surprises.

'And I've thought about whether I should tell you what I would do if you asked me again,' I said, 'because I thought you might.' That was the sort of thing I would say – 'thought you might' – like I was still wanting to think I was ahead of the game. The Master.

'And you usually don't, do you?' she said. 'I can't think of a single question you haven't got me to answer for myself.'

'Oh.' I had hoped it wasn't so obvious.

'And the way I see it, that's no accident, is it?' she said.

'No, it's no accident, Val.' It was in the manual, Reflecting Back.

'Hmm, that's what I thought. And do you know what else I've thought?' she asked.

Me, waiting.

'In the beginning I didn't think much of that way of talking to me, not answering my questions. But I've come to see that it works,' she said.

'Right, so then . . .' I started.

'So then, what would *you* do? I've thought about it, and I've run out of ideas. I just can't get Christine out of my mind. It's eating me alive.' We stopped at that one. It was a bit close to the bone.

When that seemed to settle, I said, 'I'd write a final letter.'

'A *fi*nal letter? But I've already written *plen*ty of *fi*nal letters! Christine still doesn't write back.'

'This wouldn't be written to make Christine write back,' I said. Sometimes I was tempted to speak back with the contempt and irritation she showed me. But I wasn't going to let Val decide how I was going to be. 'It would be written for you, for you to have a final say and to let that be an end to it.' She leaned back, chin up. It was her listening-while-reflecting pose. I slowed down.

'I'd write all of what I wanted to say if I had the chance to say it face to face. But the basic deal would be that if the letter wasn't responded to within a couple of weeks, I would let that be that. At least then, if I'd left nothing unsaid, I would know that I'd done all I could. There would be nothing else to be done.'

Val wrote the letter and had me post it the following week. As I let it go and heard it slide into the cold mailbox, it felt as if things were being put back in their rightful place, back into the hands of the Gods. The deadline of two weeks came and went without so much as a whisper. No surprises there. The next time I was with Val, I sat alongside her while she tore to pieces her hand-made copy of the final letter, the shreds consigned to the bin, dust to dust.

'Tea?'

That was Christine, and it seemed to leave Val smaller and weaker. She felt fragile now. She had had the courage to face up to something incomplete and uncontrollable, and had ended up a little more dismantled. Her aim was to resolve every-thing before she died, with everyone, and she had stumbled at the first post. She had to face the fact that if a final bedside reunion was going to happen, it was not going to be down to her.

She was to be distracted from her disappointment by discovering another woman even more tormented than her. On meeting this soul she suddenly found herself in the position of carer rather than patient, and this good Samaritanship extended to me by proxy. So one afternoon I arrived to find two patients waiting. Val had perked up – her friend was desolate. I got her 'patient' talking, and found her deeply despairing. I listened to her for an hour, and Val left us to it, making the tea and keeping out of our way. Seeing Val so uplifted, I couldn't help but wonder, was this what I was looking for? To be lifted out of some underlying despair? Was I being selfless? Or was I looking for an antidote to my own damage? Did it *matter* in the end? Val had helped this woman. I seemed to be helping Val. She wanted me there with her, right through to her death, she said. How selfish could that be?

MAKING FRIENDS

'You just missed my friend Sue again,' Val would sometimes say after I had slipped down into the eternally lapping foam of the oceanic sofa. She would emphasise the *my friend*. It bugged me. I think it was meant to. I was somewhere lower down the social order than *friend*. But then, Val wasn't *my* friend. I wasn't telling her about my life, my problems, my dreams. We were something else, but what that was, I wasn't sure.

'She suddenly remembered she had to be somewhere and was off!' Val said. 'No doubt you'll bump into her some day.'

Val had met Sue and Bill at bingo. 'Oh dear, you just missed Bill. I told him you'd be here any minute and the next thing I knew, he was gone.'

Sue and Bill. It would be more accurate to write 'Sue. And Bill.' In this way Sue (.) and Bill were not at all grammatical. Although they visited Val two or three times a week, it was always separately. Each occupied a distinct part of Val's sentence.

I know this only because I once bumped into Bill as he left Val's, sheepishly, by the side alley as I was arriving. I met him no more, other than in Val's mind. I knew about Sue because

Val told me about her visits, and I bumped into her once as well. Sue often left just before I arrived. As Val spoke less about Christine, she referred more and more to Sue, and Bill, telling me what they had done for her over the previous week, marvelling at their care. That they would give so much of their time affected her deeply, and was a rare redeeming feature of Val's otherwise bleak autumnal life.

Through the rejection by her daughter and the utter futility of the medical treatments, Val had managed to hold on to the love and kindness of these dear people. But, being Val, that did not mean they received the same from her. In fact she showed no sense of remorse or doubt as she acquainted me with the latest criticisms she had made about Bill to Sue, nor any feelings of responsibility for Sue's obvious discomfort on hearing them. Perhaps this was why Sue, and Bill, were not Sue and Bill in Val's life, but this in no way deterred either from their good deeds and their cherished companionship.

'Sue took me to the bank today. She's ever so nice to me.'

'Bill did the lawns already, so you won't have to do them this time.'

'Sue said she thought I ought to . . .'

'Bill told me if I wanted him to he could . . .'

'Sue rang just before you came to tell me that . . .'

I was jealous; I had to admit it. *I* was going to take Val to the bank that day; we had talked about it the week before. And *I* was going to mow the lawns, that was part of what *I* did. I was jealous; it was terrible. I had been uncomfortable for some time whenever Val mentioned Sue, and Bill, surely because I felt some tenure over Val, over her illness, over the 'opportunities' Val and her illness afforded me, a selfish self-less ownership through companionship that was being usurped by this disparate couple from somewhere down the road. I felt ashamed of myself: the juggernaut of my ego had apparently annexed the state of Val's dying.

On the other hand Val gained such comfort and felt such gratitude towards Sue, and Bill, that she went to what, for Val, was the not inconsiderable trouble of having her will altered to include them. Surveying her possessions, and excluding the house that was going to Christine 'regardless', she sought some treasure that would remember her to them. She spent some days deliberating and in the end could not quite believe her own generosity.

She rang Sue and told her she had changed the will, and did Sue want to 'pop in' to hear the decree? Yes, Sue did, and not only that but Val had the unexpected pleasure of being able to tell them both, as unusually they arrived together, at last, Sue and Bill.

Val told them she had thought about it for a long time and realised there was only one thing that would really show them how grateful she was, and thus she bequeathed them her redoubtable indomitable velour sofa (and matching arm-chairs), which would be a commanding and consoling reminder of her presence, thus helping to fill the void she would leave in their lives. If it did not replace her in essence, it surely would in volume.

When Val told me of her bequest she was clearly very pleased with herself, and we went on to talk that day about death and life after death and where, if anywhere, one goes and what about all these near-death experiences and did I know that she'd had one many years before? No, I didn't, and typically she saved that story for another time, a future time, her future.

Sue phoned Val the Thursday morning after the reading of the new will but just before I arrived at the house. Sue double-checked that I would be there on this particular day – it was the sort of consideration and kindness that warmed Val to the core. Sue told Val that she and Bill would not be visiting again, that she could not say why, and that was the last Val was going to hear from either of them. Sue put down the phone. Val stood transfixed in disbelief as tears welled in her old eyes. I walked up to her open front door to look into the lounge where she stood, still, handset in hand. I hadn't seen her shocked before. And she had had many shocks. It was awful.

Another unresolved and painfully depressing puzzle. I did not hear of Sue or Bill again. I wondered, and perhaps Val did too, whether it was because she had given too much, in terms of unsolicited and insidious advice; or too little, in terms of the sofa. Val's fate was to intertwine one final time with Bill's, as he was the fellowman at the crematorium, destined to shovel from the incinerator the dust of her mortal coil.

PLAN B
September 1994

The myeloma did not pause in sympathy for a moment at the loss of Sue or Bill. It did not falter on its inexorable way. It showed no mercy, no restraint; no accord with Val other than that of the parasite with the host.

Soon the chemotherapy treatment was completed, another box ticked: Val proudly anticipated her results. But her pride in her achievement began to dissipate into a terribly drawn-out vigil as week after week she found herself without news. This in itself was enough to resurrect her dilemma regarding her daughter – the difficulty of being without a response to her efforts being similar in both situations.

When she greeted me at the door, she said, 'I haven't heard a word.' Thus leaving it open as to whether she was referring to her daughter or the hospital or both. She would turn in, dejected.

'Why is it taking so long?' she would ask me as she eased herself down into The Great Thing. 'You'd think they could just make a telephone call, wouldn't you?' she would say as she collapsed backwards, sorrowful.

'Surely they could just call me and put me out of my misery!' But it was not only *they* she wished would put her out of her misery, for she was having a go at it as well. She had caught a chest infection and had done nothing about it, knowing full well this was exactly the sort of thing cancer patients die from, their immune system being so weakened. She was waiting to see what would happen next.

When at last the doctor did give Val The News it served only to drop her further into that misery she had hoped to be pulled out of, leaving her sinking and beleaguered rather than high and dry. She had been sure the doctors were 'right' and that the chemotherapy could and would cure her. Now that it had failed to do so, she was left with only one logical and immeasurably crushing conclusion: it was *she* who had failed, failed not only herself but all of us. To her desolation and disappointment over Christine, Sue and Bill, and the ultimately distressing force of an unknowable death, a further and condemning sense of guilt and shame was added.

Val was anxious that if she did not 'put a brave face on it', then I, like Christine, would cease to have any contact with her. Reassure her in word and presence as I might, it was inevitable that at times I would be closed out. I found such visits almost unbearable, the conversation dreadfully pleasant, as Val avoided any subject she believed might repel me.

It was not only for my benefit that Val tried to assume this 'happy' disposition; she also believed that a loss of optimism equated to a loss of life. It became for Val essential, the centre of a one-sided bargain with the Gods, to have, come what may, something to be optimistic about. And this is where the doctors unwittingly (I like to think) played an enticing hand.

According to Val, they announced an 'experimental drug' that would be ideal for her to try. She decided to undertake the treatment as it offered hope, and hope was preferable to the despair she was left in after the chemotherapy. She acknowledged that 'the doctors aren't so sure this time that this will cure me.' She was admitted to the local hospital, her worries focused on who was going to feed the new inhabitants of the pond while she was 'inside'. It was a cold autumn and the pond might soon freeze over.

I visited Val in hospital, and wondered at the appalling side effects of the drugs as they extracted her life and spirit, reducing her once more to despair but now with the constant affliction of severe nausea and searing headaches. She had not an ounce of happiness left in her and was sure on occasions that she was about to die, yet persisted with the treatment.

Val was sent home to continue the 'healing' and on a visit in late September I found her in what I took to be 'a dangerous physical state', as I had written in my visit report. Her emotional and mental states were not so hot either. I rang her nurses and doctor and concentrated my efforts on getting her into either the hospice or hospital, incensed that she had been dumped at home in such a condition. After putting down the phone, having alerted Val's doctor, I sat down beside Val. The doing was done.

'I don't know if it's worth it,' she said, referring to the 'treatment'. 'I don't have any life left at all.' She appeared remorseful, contrite, as if she were once again letting us all down, as if she was the disappointment rather than the disappointed – a mental manoeuvre children often make to reassure themselves about their failing parents.

It was odd in the assaulting overbearing décor to find her so subdued and defenceless. 'If this is going to be how it is then I think I'd rather not keep going,' she said, sounding like a young girl, pressed into the side of the sofa, depressed, cornered.

'Had you expected any of this?' I asked, rather pointlessly. I couldn't see that her answer would make any difference, unless I was going to say 'Then it serves you right!' Either way, expect it or not, she would have chosen the experimental drugs.

'No, not really. They said I might feel a bit fluey, that was all. But it's far worse than a *bit fluey*! I just feel so dreadful all the time. I mean it's not a *life*, is it?'

God, it was an awful moment. 'No, it's not much of a life, Val,' I said, feeling such admiration for this courageous woman, aware of how petty I could be in my own little mediocre world. The feeling of being powerless was infectious, but it was much more than a feeling, it was the actuality: life being so completely out of our hands. We didn't much like it.

After a few minutes of quiet she said, 'I think I have to stop the drugs, Paul; it's just too much for me.' She breathed out a relieving sigh. 'It's just such an awful way to be alive.' And I saw her body appear to cave in, only half an inch, but significantly cave in. 'I feel like they've used me as some sort of guinea-pig. Who cares about some old woman who's going to die anyway?'

The air was cold on the ride home, and the motorway ahead was empty. I checked my mirror, the lanes behind were pretty empty as well, just pairs of yellow dots way back, zig-zagging insanely in the vibrating mirror. 'Potato-potato-potato,' said my Harley. I twisted the throttle back, how I loved that sound, and potatoed up to ninety-five. Smooth. Just gliding along. But the force of the air on me was tremen-dous. Especially when I stood up on the foot-pegs and started screaming. I could barely hold on. But there was much more screaming to do. And you've no idea how frightening it was, how hard to hold on to the hand-grips, when I put my boots on the seat, and crouched there. Ninety-five miles per hour, on a cold September night. When the stars were the starriest stars I'd ever seen, I surfed a motorway in England.

HOME
October 1994

Another twist, another turn, no stable ground for Val, no caravanserai in which she could pitch her tent for a night; only sandstorms and a continually changing landscape. She liked it in the hospice now and her spirits began to lift, and this in turn began to affect her physical health. She began to look more alive and lively as I visited her there. One afternoon as I squeaked my rubber-soled way down the silent corridors I was accosted by one of the hospice doctors. He told me something unexpected had happened. The pattern in a person dying of myeloma was for their white blood cell count to diminish until they died, but in Val's case the pattern was, at this point at least, inexplicably reversing.

'There's more for Val to do,' I thought, but I was wrong; I should have said there was more for Val to *find*. When I had first met Val she had a prognosis of death within one to three months; we were together for eighteen months in all. It's a puzzle.

Improving health and disposition brought Val to what was for her the regrettable point of earning a ticket out of the hospice; the bed was needed for someone more desperate. She had by this time moved from 'a fear and trembling' of hospices as places from which you only checked out wearing a wooden kimono, to an experience of a safe institutionalised haven, of expert and interested carers who met not only her physical needs but also her yearning for companionship at any time of day or night, for fellow awareness of her existence. From this calm harbour Val was instructed to return to the otherwise empty house that she had thought she had left in her wake. She had become a little boat moored to a wharf only to be sent out to sea again, as if she was still the ship she once had been. Thus she experienced her progress not as a reprieve but as a sentence to the loneliness and despair of a previous existence.

Her response was common for patients in such a predicament, that of trepidation at having to leave the cosseted warmth and attention of the hospice, the hospital, the institution, in much the same way that a long-term prisoner might fear their own freedom. Afraid, she asked repeatedly if it was not possible for her to stay; she wasn't 'much trouble after all'. But the bed was needed; she could not refuse to go. The nurses phoned me to ask if I could take Val back home. When I arrived, thick with motorway smog, I found her sitting dejected beside the bed that was no longer hers. It was a dismal sight. She looked as though she thought she had done something wrong, by getting better. I could see it in her face: 'I'm sorry. I didn't mean to. It's not fair. Why do I always have to end up on my own?'

I wondered how this unwelcome parole might affect her. I remembered how disorienting and depressing it had been for me several years before when I had, to the amazement of doctors and family, survived a disease that by all accounts should have killed me. My initial reward was to be ejected from the asylum of hospital to convalesce and depress alone for several weeks in a dilapidated old house, bewildered and unprepared. I spent many lonely days in that echoing building in immobilised melancholic confusion: the doldrums.

We pulled up in Val's driveway in my dogged little car and sat silently together in the diminishing warmth. We remained there for several minutes before Val ventured out of that shared space, in the knowledge that soon I would leave her, alone for the first time in weeks, weeks she had wrongly gauged to be the entire remainder of her life. There would soon be no one to talk to and no one to listen. No one to help her to the loo, to fetch her a cup of tea, to fluff her pillows, or even to glance in recognition as she lay securely anchored in the bay of their care. She put a stoic face on it, being Val, which made the situation all the more heartrending. I offered to sleep over that first night, but she was too proud to accept.

Val was experiencing, in the heightened way the dying can, the sort of soulless dissociation many experience on returning home from school, the office, the supermarket, the affair; when they come face to face with what they have settled for at the cost of their souls – a safe cage at the cost of their freedom. The difference being that Val *knew* she was experiencing it.

'How about making us a cup of tea, Paul?' she said.

So there it was, the capitulation, the deafening declaration of her defeat. I trudged off to the kitchen, my captain mortally wounded on her ship. In solitude, biting back the tears, I performed Val's Way of Tea.

The house looked cold and empty from the outside and was precisely that on the inside. Val walked tentatively around the lounge, picking things up, putting them gently down, as if she were a bored explorer who had stumbled upon an insignificant tomb. There was a curtain now between who she had become and who she had been, and she pondered on how any of these things could have meant anything to her at any time. She had walked into a life that was now almost totally meaningless to her, and had been told that it was hers, that she had to stay.

LIFELINE

The visits to Val took on an intensity beyond anything I had previously experienced with her. She became immersed in the persuasive and pervasive sense that although she was 'doing well' her time was running out. I arrived one afternoon to hear that her Lifeline – a white plastic amulet sporting a red panic button, which hung around her neck – had 'given up the ghost'.

'I'm supposed to keep it with me all the time,' she said. 'All I have to do is push the button and someone will come right over and pick me up or put me down or roll me over or do whatever it is I can't do that needs doing. But it's gone dead, Paul. I don't have a lifeline any more.' She just looked at me in the hope that somewhere in the dim recesses of my cerebral cavity I might Get It.

With that she slowly steamed to the kitchen to make Tea. On some visits everything that needed to be said was said in a few words. What was to be thought and felt and contemplated from those words could go on for hours and days, even years. There was little time to assimilate as the cancer in her effortlessly accelerated, down hill, towards a complete standstill. And then, in destroying its host, in cutting off its nose to spite its face, the cancer would destroy itself.

Rummaging through the dark garage looking for something for Val later that day, I happened upon an old photographic enlarger lying neglected and dusty in a rotting cardboard box. Having salvaged what Val had sent me for, I mentioned this extra find on my return, revealing one of the legion of my unsavoury facets, covetousness. When I was blessed with childhood and cursed with Catholicism, I knew, having heard the commandment Thou Shalt Not Covet Thy Neighbour's Goods, that my soul was in peril. I was pretty sure I could make it with the other nine, even the coveting wives thing – not quite knowing what it was as a boy, I was sure if it had anything to do with grown-ups it must be dreadfully dull. But the goods issue was surely going to keep me out of their heaven. I could not help it. I had grown up on hand-me-downs from my older brother and so became accustomed to view what he had as soon-to-be-mine. This view spread to include other people's goods. It must have been *how* I said it because Val *knew* I wanted it.

The thing was, I didn't. I was just coveting. I did the coveting, I could have done without the attaining. But I could tell, by how she looked, that she was already planning to give the enlarger to me. I knew that I would not be able to say 'No thanks' gracefully, even though once I had the thing it would feel wrong to get rid of it. And she did give it to me, and it did all feel terribly wrong.

Her life seemed a mess, a God-awful mess, and it was all too easy to get caught up in it. Any weakness in me left me vulnerable to being sucked into any eddy created by the greater flow. And this one I was sucked into, this gift became a part of the swansong Val was conceiving for herself, although ultimately her end was to be an altogether inconceivable one.

ME!

Val began to settle in at home again, but there was a tepid atmosphere, a hopelessness in her house. She couldn't help but notice, on going back, that her life had been ordinary. She said so, which is how I know. She realised she had settled for mediocrity, and could no longer pretend, only go through the motions like a traffic light: go – doubt – stop – doubt – go …

We talked without need of direction or resolution, once for six hours straight, about life, beans, the universe, toilet flush mechanisms, tennis, God and everything.

She had begun to sieve through the *Rubaiyat* of Omar Khayyam, given 'To Val, Wishing you a very happy Xmas, With love from Tom'. Now I would come gently through the unlocked doorway of her house to find Val ensconced on the rejected sofa, the *Rubaiyat* rifled and revealed at her side, she ruminating on the numerous 'puzzles' Khayyam served up:

> *Oh, come with old Khayyam, and leave the Wise*
> *To talk; one thing is certain, that Life flies;*
> *One thing is certain, and the Rest is Lies;*
> *The Flower that once has blown forever dies.*

'Do you think we have more than one life?' Val would gnaw away at this contentious bone for hours, by herself and with me. Her spiritual life had been utterly impoverished and her suspicions that I was a theist led us into many searching conversations. I said nothing about my experiences or perspective, wanting neither to alienate her from her atheism nor to throw her into an imagined collusive religiosity in which her doubts and questions might sink without trace. I once sat with a priest who was dying; he was no longer sure there was God. I doubt he had ever been closer to Him, nor He to him.

There were always those who could be summoned – priest, vicar, rabbi, monk, psychoanalyst, scientist – delighted to summarily execute the patient's reservations regarding this tricky issue of life after death. Any one of them, caught up in their books, could put Val straight regarding this question of God by introducing their own, from Buddha to The Second Law of Thermodynamics to Freud. She knew and I knew that all she had to do was to ask if it was indeed an answer she wanted. It was the question itself she needed. More than any answer it reflected who and where and what Val was. She had reached on her own merit the very same place as Heidegger when he said the relation of any human being to the world is that of a question. She had no use for anyone else's answer; she had only her right to be in the question, to not know, to be unsure. The definite were of no interest to her, only the interested, the compassionately curious, those able to risk, if only for a single hour.

There is one visit to her house engraved into me like no

other, when one harsh winter day I arrived to find Val in a most epiphanous state. Quietly but urgently she drew me in and sat me down. The *Rubaiyat* was open on the table with tiny notes sticking out of it on pieces of blue-lined white paper. There was no immediate 'Tea?!' which could only mean one thing: something was up.

With an unexpected excitement, she said, 'I've got something really important to tell you. I've been waiting to tell you because I couldn't tell anyone else, they wouldn't Get It. But I think you will.'

I was beginning to believe in love again. I waited. This was what Val had begun to remind me of, the root of everything.

'I was standing in the kitchen,' she began, sitting as if alone in the room, face searching ahead to nowhere, hands resting upturned on her trousered lap. 'I was making myself something that I knew I'd never eat, but I thought it was important to go to the bother of doing it anyway. So I did.

'I was making a little roast: some potatoes and some beans, and a nice bit of chicken that Maureen got for me from up the road.' She turned conspiratorially to add, 'Why she would waste her money there I don't know, they're very expensive. Still, it's her money, and if she wants to throw it away it's got nothing to do with me, I suppose.'

She turned back into her reverie, 'And then suddenly I just stopped.' She paused for breath and seemed to look deep within to find the experience once more. 'The kitchen knife was in my hand, in mid-air,' she held up her right hand, 'and I just stopped.' This she did as I watched from my different time zone two feet away. 'I didn't move for I don't know how long. It might have been a minute, it might have been an hour, I don't know, but I knew that time didn't matter. And Paul,' her arm dropped slowly as she turned to face me, aglow, 'while I was standing there I realised something, something I hadn't realised before. I said to myself, "I'm not Val". It was wonderful. So peaceful. I said, "I'm not Val. I'm not an old woman. I'm not this and I'm not that. I'm just me. I'M. ME! And I *love* it!"' And at that she managed with a sharp upward celebratory thrust of her arms to momentarily free herself from the gravitational pull of the black hole that was the sofa, before falling back down into it.

'And I haven't felt the same since!' she said.

Val sat back flushed, happy and magnificent. *Alterius non sit, qui suus esse potest.* Be not another if thou canst be thyself. And at that point I realised I loved her and didn't want her to die, and that I hadn't thought any of this was going to happen.

We sat there, two pilgrims. We were silent for a long while, maybe a minute, maybe an hour, I do not know. Time did not matter. We gazed out intrepid and hopeful from the enterprising craft that was Val's sofa, out to the grey bay of her decaying garden and far beyond to the dark unfathomable oceans of the world. Christmas was coming, and it would be Val's last.

The weather drew us in. A dull and permanent Tupperware lid of cloud shut out the sky and shut in a drizzle-drenched England, as Val and I headed towards a second Christmas together. The hedge had been cut one last time, the lawn no longer needed mowing, the leaves had pretty much all fallen. Val was gradually becoming more accepting of the *fact* that she was dying but didn't accept that she would actually die.

She continued to talk of her garden in terms of crops and flowers in the years to come, confident that she would make it to the spring of the following year. Yet she would often signal the end of such a train of thought by looking at me with a little knowing smile, perhaps happy that she had been granted a collusive reprieve from facing her decline and demise.

An aspect of Val's defence against death lay in the reassurance of food, a defence often shored up by her infrequent visitors. Sitting in the hospice or hospital wards, the most common greeting I would hear given to patients by family or friends was, 'Hello, So-and-so, you're looking well!'

Thus the visitor brings into question the authenticity of the patient's claim for a sick-bed, in the same stroke abandoning them to the lonely vigil over the progression of their illness, while making it clear that they, the healthy visitor, intend to maintain only a temporary and marginal presence. Having dug in, the visitor advances along the second prong of, let's face it, attack: 'Have you been eating properly?'

Have you eaten? Did you have a good breakfast/lunch/dinner? You look as though you've put on some weight! These are such common questions, statements, attributes and injunctions, regardless of the state of the patient, and usually put with such haste that it appears reasonable to assume the visitor is making an attempt to establish something of significance. The logic is simple, and was expounded by Val one day when she said, 'Well, at least I can't die as long as I eat every day.'

It seemed extraordinary to me at the time that an intelligent person could believe such a thing, and even more so that it made little difference to her if that 'something' was a roast dinner or a single crisp. It was food and so enabled and ensured life to her but, as we headed for Christmas, Val's appetite dwindled to a spoonful of soup rather than half a chicken.

On the first day of December 1994, Val and I drove out to the local garden centre. Val was most anxious about not being able to control the car, her tiny feet frantically hunting the floor in vain for some sign of brake or accelerator (I was driving). To get out of the house was a real treat for her, and for me a welcome respite from that oppressive low-ceilinged tomb. Beyond telling me how to drive, Val sat enthroned and satisfied.

We wandered round the centre looking at the plants and

flowers and then sat, the *puer eternus* and the *sennex*, in the little café. I was about to go abroad for five weeks, leaving her in a subdued despondency over the disintegration of her health, life and relationships, and a determined will to live as fully as possible during the time granted.

'I've died before, you know,' said Val. 'It was during an operation. I was under general anaesthetic and my heart stopped beating. I can remember it clearly! I was looking down at the theatre staff as if I was floating six feet over their heads. I could see myself lying on the operating table, and I wondered what all the fuss was about. I didn't know I was dead. It didn't cross my mind that I shouldn't have been up in the air and lying on the operating table at the same time. I just couldn't understand what all the excitement was about.' She smiled.

'Then I felt this mighty *thump!* in my chest, and the next thing I knew I was waking up in the hospital bed the next day. I told the surgeon what had happened, the floating in the air and seeing myself lying there and the thump in my chest. And he said, "That must have been when we gave your heart an electric shock." I looked down under my nightdress and there were two big purple bruises, right on my chest.'

My report of the day says that at the garden centre we had 'a long and deep discussion about levels of consciousness, the spirit and what happens after death'. For someone who had done away with the Gods, existing after her death had left quite an impression on Val. She had no formal framework to hang it on, but this did not stop her talking about things like the soul, reincarnation, the nature of awareness,

identity, self, and many things that I, in my conceit, had not
expected to discuss with her. She was changing. Or she was
coming out of hiding. 'I'm me! And I love it.'

We bought a large Christmas tree that day, and Val booked
me to decorate it the following week. The tree leaned menacingly against the wall in Val's lounge, tap root cut, an open
challenge for Val to make it to Christmas.

ASCENSION

When I arrived at Val's home seven days later, I found the tree already gaudily bedecked and bejewelled. The decorations had been stored in the attic – I knew this because I was supposed to retrieve them that very day – but there they were, perched audaciously on the tree in unambiguous defiance of any sense of taste, bar that of Las Vegas at midnight.

'So who got the decorations down for you?' I asked, knowing it could not have been Sue. Or Bill.

'Not who, *how*!' Val replied, triumphant. I wondered if her euphoria was pharmacological or psychological, but joined in regardless.

'How?' I repeated.

Val nodded and said, 'It's a puzzle. You figure it out and tell me when you think you've got it. Tea?!'

The attic was entered through a small trap door in a nine-foot-high ceiling. 'Did you climb up there?' I asked.

'Well I didn't *fly* up there!' she said. Enjoying ourselves, we were.

'You climbed up by yourself?' I said.

'Of course by myself.' She leaned back and said, 'I wasn't

about to carry anyone *else* up there, was I?' Happy, having a good time.

In the intervening week she had had another blood transfusion. As usual the revivifying blood suffused her with enough dynamism to go for twenty-four hours without sleep, at a time when she was usually sleeping away three-quarters of each of her remaining days. Fuelled by the plasma-drive, she had dragged an aluminium ladder from the garage to the house, and then pulled it up the stairs by sitting on each step in turn like some incapacitated but fanatical mountain climber. She established base camp at the crest of the stairs, then erected the ladder under the porthole in the ceiling. She climbed precariously but valiantly into the attic, in the knowledge that the highly probable fall would highly probably kill her.

Val was experiencing her life as having a whole new range of possibilities, many of the previous ones having been decimated by the cancer.

Her disease, multiple myeloma, is caused by the rampant uncontrolled growth of plasma cells within the marrow of one's bones, and these cells produce an antibody that cannot fight infection. As if that were not enough, they produce substances that can dissolve your bones, particularly the spine, the pelvis, the rib cage, and the skull.

So our intrepid hero, Val, seated on the ceiling, was susceptible at any time to skeletal problems (solitary or multiple osteolytic lesions, diffuse osteoporosis), bone destruction (elevated serum calcium, hypercalcuria, loss of height), extra-skeletal myeloma (soft tissue problems, mostly around the head and neck but possibly also the liver, kidneys, and other soft tissue), peripheral blood problems (anaemia, abnormal clotting, leucopenia, plasma cell leukaemia, circulating monoclonal B lymphocytes), plasma protein changes (hyperproteinaemia, hypervolaemia, monoclonal immunoglobins, amyloidosis, narrowed anion gap, elevated serum B20 microglobulin, decreased serum albumin, elevated serum IL6 and C-reactive protein) and kidney problems (proteinuria, casts without leucocytes or erythrocytes, tubular dysfunction with acidosis, uraemia – kidney failure).

What these could do to her, sitting there, waiting, is bring about pain of varying intensity, often in the lower back or ribs, severe pain in the case of fracture or vertebral collapse, general malaise, bruising, nose bleeding, hazy vision, headaches, gastrointestinal bleeding, loss of appetite, nausea, vomiting, thirst, passing out, swollen ankles, breathing difficulties, bacterial infection, fevers, shivering, sleepiness and exhaustion brought about by reduced blood and oxygen supply to the nerve tissue, spinal chord compression, and meningitis.

To try to manage these symptoms, but not the myeloma itself, Val could face treatment through chemotherapy, highdose therapy with transplant, radiation, alpha interferon, erythropoietin, bisphosphonates, dialysis, plasmapheresis, pain medication, antibiotics, growth hormones, brace, corset, exercise, diet, and new drugs.

Then, in order to try to monitor all of this – the disease, the pathophysiology, the treatments – Val could also be subject to regular testing which might include blood counts, chemistry panel, liver function tests, M protein measurements, serum B microglobulin, C-reactive protein, peripheral blood labelling index, serum erythropoietin level, routine urinanalysis, 24-hour urine tests for Bence Jones protein and albumin plus creatinine clearance, skeletal survey using x-rays to evaluate bones, MRI/CT scan for special problems, other scans if required, bone density measurement, bone marrow aspiration and biopsy for diagnosis and periodic monitoring and special testing to assess prognosis, plus other testing depending upon special circumstances such as amyloidosis, neuropathy, renal and infectious complications.

So her venture to the attic, and to her own interior, was to my mind an act of pure heroism. I salute her. Having summited, she sat exhausted for an hour in the light of a bare bulb. She was like some astonished Edmund Hillary, waiting for his breathing to return to normal before taking the usual photographs. She rallied enough borrowed strength to drag the large box of decorations, atheistically labelled XMAS, to the edge of the porthole. And there she rested again, in the quiet solitude of altitude.

Descent is often more precarious than ascent. And, unusually for a climber, Val was taking down more gear than she had taken up. She had pulled the box out over the edge of the hole, and climbed down the ladder to where her head was level with the base of the box. She pulled the box out over the lip, and balanced it on her head while leaning it against the rails of the ladder. Now more Sherpa Tenzing than Hillary, she had slowly descended the ladder with the box sliding down on the rails above her.

'The rest', she said, 'was child's play.'

On 22 December I saw Val again. She believed she was growing inside. I believed I was too, but I said nothing about that.

'It's not what I'd expected,' she said. 'And I think it's got something to do with you.' She looked across to me from her end of the sofa, 'Is that right?'

'How do you mean?' I asked.

'When I was told I had cancer I thought that was it. That nothing good could possibly come out of it. But now I'm not so sure. I think a lot of good might come out of it. What do you think?'

'What good?'

'Well, I quite like being me now. I'm doing a bit more reading, and I'm really thinking about things.' She looked over to her *Rubaiyat*. 'I'll read something, like this,' and she leaned forward to pick the book up off the table. She could not do it, her stomach was too round and firm. Steroids. I did not interfere. She had to get up to reach the book, and then she sat down again, and opened the book to a page with a piece of paper sticking out of it. She read what she had written on the paper:

*There was a door
to which I found no
key*

'And that's it, you see, Paul. I've thought about this one for days. Because I've had this feeling, that I think I may have found the key. I think *I* could be the key. And that's a new thing for me to think about myself, a new way to see myself. It's what I meant about what happened in the kitchen that day. Do you see what I mean?'

'Yes.'

'And,' she sifted through the red hardback again, until she found another slip of paper. She read it to me, her glasses on her nose:

The wine of life keeps oozing drop by drop, The leaves of life keep falling one by one.

'And that's exactly what it's been like, Paul. "Drop by drop" and "one by one". That's how everything seems to be going. I keep thinking about this one too. They're all like puzzles. They look small, but in fact they're really huge. I don't much like it, losing things and people, even drop by drop. And some people could have been much kinder to me about things. But it doesn't hurt so much now. Not *now*. It just seems like it has to be that way, and there's nothing I or anybody else can do about it. "Drop by drop." I quite like that idea.

'At least I've got the time to let go of things, drop by drop. It would be terrible just to get run over or shot or something. And I'd never have thought of it before all this, but in a way I'm luckier than some. I can try to put some things right, get things in order, before I go. It's not so bad, is it?'

Val put the slip back into the *Rubaiyat*, from where it had come, and flicked through until she found a third. Same procedure, she read it in her own hand:

Think then you are
today what yesterday
you were —
Tomorrow you shall
not be less

'I've only begun to really work on this one. It's what's called a Par A Dox.' She looked into me, as if she was trying to see whether her words had hit a target in there. *Thock!*

'Not the words themselves, but what's happening to me. I can see that I'm dying, piece by piece. There's no denying that. But what's very odd is that I don't feel any less. It's almost like I feel I'm *more* than I was before. If that makes any sense.'

And so she went on, back and forth through her *Rubaiyat*. Her book of puzzles. Her health that day was surprisingly good, and under the tree she had me find a little present and a card. I hadn't bought her anything. I would bring something back with me from New Zealand. But I hadn't even given her so much as a card. I was still too caught up in the training I'd had. Just to be human, God what I'd give for that!

'Shall I open it now?'

'Do you always open your presents before Christmas!?' she said.

I waited.

My final visit before going away was a week later. I felt a little better about leaving because she was in relatively good health and spirits. I wrote that I was worried 'that the good health is too good to be true (my fear) and that I will not see her again for another five weeks (Val's fear)'. When I left her that day, I had no doubts about her will or determination – the tree was testimony to that. What bothered me was that these 'strengths' could become the very obstacles to her having a peaceful death. But then, who said her death had to be peaceful? Or my life?

She walked me to the front door as usual, and as we said goodbye we both knew it could be for good. There were no guarantees. There were no stakes in the ground. There was no ground outside of what was in us. A bond had grown between us, through error and trial over the preceding year. And this was silently recognised, when Val stepped forward to hug me. It was warm. She was small and weak, but held me as firmly as a child's fist holds your little finger. She reached up and pulled my head down a little, so she could kiss my cheek. It wasn't sentimental, we just didn't know how much of a goodbye we were making. We were going to miss each other, really miss each other, and this was throwing us both. I flew out that night.

I carried Val within me in New Zealand. Not being with her, or arranging my week around seeing her, made me realise what a huge part of my life she had become. I thought about her every day. I wondered if she was still alive. I felt bonded to her, right through the middle of the earth. I would sit – bare feet, shorts, a wide-brimmed cotton hat – surrounded by waving sea grasses on a warming dune. And my heart would fill with Val, left behind in the diminished light of a bitterly cold England.

Part Three

World Without End

DROWNING
1964

When I was six I gave up the idea of learning to swim. I gave it up because I was terrified of the swimming coach. One morning he held my head under water because he was angry about my not breathing 'properly'. Of course I panicked. With his hand around the back of my neck I tried to scream, but that made it worse when the water shot into my throat. He kept me under until things started going black, as if he hated me, then stars appeared. Then he let me go. But I was so frightened I could not move and he had to jerk my head out of the water. He was furious. I thought he was going to hold me under again, and I started to cry. My brother, John, was right beside me. I felt so ashamed. The instructor told me to 'Get out!' I got out. I couldn't stop shaking while I got dressed in the cold changing room. Who *are* these people?

When I got home I had to tell my Dad what happened, because he asked me how swimming went. I did not want him to know I was such a little weakling. But then John took my side. And when he did this, which he never did, I knew what the coach did must have been really bad. Dad went down to the pool to have A Word with him. But the next week, Dad left me there again, with that man. I could not believe it. I didn't learn to swim. I was too afraid to put my head under the water, any water. Even in the shower I could begin to panic. I did not tell anyone this, I kept quiet.

1977

Thirteen years later I was about to enrol for the third year of my psychology degree. I woke one summer's morning to a warm, plump, deep-blue promising day. Everything, even I, felt essential.

My brother John drove us north out of town towards Maori Bay. Heady odours of humid freshly mown grass and hot tar seal wafted in through the open windows of the car. Our long hair blew around like silk scarves. We were young, we were beautiful, and we were brave. John's car was from some Eastern Bloc country, so spares were scarce and relia-bility almost non-existent. The car had a nickname. We were at that age when cars were companions. They needed us. The relationship was one of patient sacrifice, just to keep the car on the road. I don't remember the car's name, but I do remember that the sound of it made you want to be gentle and sympathetic. And anyway, you had to have a rubbish car to be a *real* surfer.

The back seat was covered with bottles of water, jostling around to see which would be next to be fed to the ever thirsty radiator. On the rusty roof were two surfboards flap-ping in linen board bags our mother had sewn for us. It must have been a breezy day, because we couldn't have gone fast enough to generate any turbulence of our own. We were followed by a long train of attentive cars, as we made slow progress out of town. We were headed towards sand dunes, brown bikini'd girls, and ruthless surging seas.

In the car I was, as usual, sneaking glances through the top of the windscreen. I could not help myself, I had to keep checking that the surfboards hadn't fallen off. I didn't want to be seen to be anxious – we were brave. And there the boards always were, annoyingly. All that checking, for all those years. If they had come off just *once*, I would have been right to worry, I wouldn't have been paranoid.

But I had greater reasons to be scared by the time I was seventeen. I no longer believed in the Gods. They had forgotten me, hadn't watched over me like They were supposed to. I had thrown out the Church, and made the mistake of throwing out the Gods at the same time. I was alone.

To the relief of all those following us in their boiling cars, we finally arrived at the beach. I had been warned about the surf there, a strong rip by the rocks on the left-hand side. 'Just make sure you stay well away from the rocks on the left,' John told me. I walked into the water, absolutely foaming. 'Who the *Hell* does he think he *is*? Does he think I've never surfed before, or something?' I paddled out furiously, to the left, through the breaking surf and then sat on my board, with its painted red and orange flames, and waited, watching the swell. It's amazing how it calms you down. I floated there, checking out the horizon, or watching the hairs on my brown legs swirling about in the clear water.

There is always a wave that catches your attention out of

all the fuzzy lines way out. It might lift up a little, as if it's trying to make you notice it. This is the one, it looms in, while the others are just there. It might seem more alive than the others, more hopeful. It's like a huge approaching snake, slithering sideways, silent and awesome, closing in on you. Then suddenly it's right there. I saw my wave and was caught. I turned towards the beach and paddled as hard as I could. Paddled, paddled, then lifted into the clear, blue, hurtling velocity. The sound of spray was loud and close behind me as my board cut into the green glass. I crouched low, perfectly balanced on my board like a t'ai chi master. Fan. Tas. Tic. Then suddenly nothing beneath my feet, the water is where the sky should be, and I'm thrown into an appalling dis-equilibrium.

I lost my surfboard on the rocks, and was sucked down into the tightening, churning sea. Salt water drove deep into my ears and tried to explode my sinuses. The sea tore at my wetsuit and ground me into the sand. It tumbled my body around like a washing machine and yanked at my limbs with an incredible force. But worst of all, I was under the water, tons of water and I couldn't get up to the surface, to the air. Held down by the giant hand of God. I had come off my board many times so I knew this was something far more serious than usual. Experience told me to wait, to wait for the pressure to let me go so I could begin to rise to the surface. Frightened, I waited. Waited.

Bubbles and sand curled around my body. 'Fuck!' I wasn't rising. 'Stupid, stupid bastard!' I was in trouble. I could feel it. My body knew about these things. 'Relax, relax.' I was being dragged along the sandy bottom on my back. I tried to turn over so I could grab something. I couldn't. The huge movement of water out of that small bay sucked me downwards and out to sea. Suddenly my hand scraped against a rock, and instinctively I grabbed at it and took a hold. I began to climb towards the surface, hanging on to the rock like a flag on a windy day. Except there was no air there. It took so much strength to climb, to break through to the air, to breathe.

One pure succulent gulp of full living air, as I glanced to my right I saw, no more than fifty yards away, a group of strong tanned surfers lolling on their boards in the reassuring sunshine. They dismissed the waves that were drowning me as not worth riding. Somewhere in that group was my brother. But in that second I was above the surface no one turned to see me, as I took a second breath to fill my lungs to yell. Engulfed by a breaking wave, I was sucked spiralling down. Not again, please, no. He was holding me under, again, I knew He would.

Rocks obscured in bubbles and sand spun around me as I reached out again and again. The rocks were just *there*, the other surfers were just a shout away, and an infinity of air was no more than twelve feet above me, with hot cars in the car park and people on the beach worrying at their ice creams as they dripped down their sandy sticky hands. And I was just over *here*, and no one knew, and no one there had any idea what it was like to be me over here, and that was my life.

The panic was the worst. It lived in the water itself. It

forced its way into me and pulled and tugged from the inside. I was getting weak, and the weaker I became the more frightened I became, until there was no Paul left, only a pure unimpaired horror, as the rest of you breathed contentedly close by.

I became so exhausted and stricken I could not move my arms at all; grabbing and climbing were no longer possible. I was overcome by disbelief that this could be happening to me. I was utterly desolate, utterly defeated, even my mind began to flee the dreadful predicament the rest of me would have to suffer to the end. I started to wonder what would happen in the life I was now about to leave, clear that death held me now, free to surrender and let myself be held.

My girlfriend would be very angry. She had told me never to surf at '*that* beach'. And my brother, floating above my new world like a cloud warming himself in the sunshine, he would surely Get It from mum. I began to imagine my funeral, hoping many people would gather to pay their last respects. But most of all I longed for them to be, if not inconsolably bereft, at least more than a little sad. For that would mean the most important thing of all: that I had loved and been loved. To me this was the most consoling possibility when all other possibilities had sunk.

All systems closed down. Even the desolation was gone. I was gone, elsewhere, commended to the forces beyond me. There were no thoughts or memory of where I had been that instant or lifetime before. Elsewhere was life itself, a welcoming reassuring glow that was at once familiar yet alien. Elsewhere curved smoothly, membranously in front of 'me'. I felt found, home. There was perfect peace, no contention. I moved forward to have a look. At the same moment, out of the corner of my awareness I sensed an indistinct pathway and an indistinct presence. I turned towards them without effort, then – BANG – I was returned to the surface.

Theseasaltysilkythebluebluesaltysea and a hard suck of the air,
thecloudssosoamazingwhitewhite, a hard suck of air,
icantouchitsobluesobluesoskysky, suck on the air,
ohmyarmsinthewatermylegs, suck it,
Godcoldsocold, suck it in,
i'mherei'mhere,
a big breath,
a whisper,
'I'm here.'

My surfboard floated beside me like a loyal dog, resigned to itself while I had been fooling around under the water. My chest heaved as the lolling, gentle sea supported my body rising and falling, rising and falling. Every tiny pore of my skin could feel that sea, the whole of it. I managed to pull myself onto my board and slowly paddle away from the rocks, towards my brother. 'I'm over here, John.' I could see him clearly because the sea had become completely calm. As I inched along the panic began to rise in me again. I heard a wounded animal bellow, 'JOHN! I'M HERE!' *That* got his attention. He turned and acknowledged me with an implied roll of his eyes. It didn't matter. I didn't care. I waited, lost in the quivering blueness of that sky, in the irresistible skyness of that sky, in the overpowering ocean-ness of that ocean. It was all too brutal an assault to experience at one time. I'd just been born, fully cognitive and sensate and unblunted.

John was soon *here*, paddling along behind me. He pushed my board ahead each time he caught up, trying to help me catch a small wave in the rebuilding surf. Oh how I loved my brother then, I would have died for him. I was lifted by a small helpful wave, propelled forward on my flaming board, reincarnating. It was a long way in, a long way from elsewhere. I dropped to my knees on the solid sand and I couldn't believe I was there, that it was real. My body trembled. I stood and walked up the beach a little, turned back towards the sea, and plonked down on the sand. I shuddered to my marrow on that hot sunny day. It was an epiphany just to watch the blood mix with sand and salt water on my cut knee. I basked in the stinging pain of the ends of my fingers, made raw from the rasping rocks. John continued to surf, and good on him. What was I going to tell him, anyway? I wasn't even sure I was willing to know myself. Where had I been? Had it happened? Is that what it is like to die? Is this what it is like to really be alive?

Now I was back. I had not been forgotten after all. I wondered if the sand went all the way to the centre of the earth. I lay back. It felt as if it did. I lay there squinting up at the solid deep blue sky. There were stars up there, all the time, moving at unimaginable speed. You just couldn't see them right now, but they were always there. Some things are like that. Me, drowning, was like those stars, always there, but hidden. And other things were too: Samantha lying on the road, Dad flat out on the porch, had also become stars for me, things that happened too far away to see, except at night when it was dark and there was nothing else – and I tried to make sure that didn't happen.

I lay on the sand that went all the way to the centre of the earth. The stars above me were always there and we lay there, all of us, bound by Gods and eternity and we knew. We could feel it.

RETURN
2 February 1995

While I was away, another volunteer visited Val. In her first report she wrote:

She was pleased to see me but was having her first 'bad day' for a while – cold and no energy ... I made us both a cup of coffee – Val hates having to let someone do things for her ... she spoke at length about her treatment – she has been having injections of a new drug – it had made her very sick and she had called out the doctor and really thought she would die. She said she is not afraid of dying – only of dying alone ... she also mentioned a pain in her shoulder, 'I hope it's not the lymphoma coming back'. Does she believe/hope it's gone? ... I am concerned about her eating – she doesn't always want a proper meal – 'Not every day'.

And in a later report, the volunteer added:

Val is in Frimley Park (Hospital) – I sat and listened to her. Sad at the deterioration of Val's health – she has had a blood transfusion which she says has not had the

same effect as a previous one – she is frustrated at feeling
so tired and sleeping as much as she is. She feels the
doctors are doing nothing and not telling her anything
. . . she wants to be in control and she can't. Val spoke
of her fear that her death is getting nearer and she's not
ready – she knows it is inevitable but has 'small things'
she wants/needs to do at home to prepare. Fears are that
the treatment has had no effect and that this is the
myeloma coming back 'to get me'. Val was quite low,
for her, and apologising for complaining – I reassured
her and tried to encourage her to continue complaining
– which she did.

Val finds it very difficult being imprisoned.

Val's myeloma was more than a disease, it was a presence,
an entity, a being with a mind and a purpose of its own that
Val was forced to share her cells with. Myeloma was ruth-
lessly and malevolently setting about the absolute destruction
of everything in Val's life that mattered, and everything that
did not, including Val. Myeloma was going to ensure she lost
everything. It would not waver in the task, would have no
mercy, no reservations, would not be defeated. Myeloma was
gradually taking over every single aspect of her life from the
most irrelevant to the most essential, from the inside out.
Forever and ever. Amen. I had not left Val alone; I had left
her with myeloma.

Not one day passed while I was away that I did not worry
and wonder whether Val was alive or dead. As soon as I was
back in London and through my front door, I was on the

phone, trying to get hold of her. There was no answer. I rang repeatedly, because if a soap opera was on the TV she would not be answering the telephone. Still, nothing. That meant I would have to try the other places she could be. But I didn't want to. I wanted Val to be at home, and OK, and waiting for me with mild disinterest because she was feeling so good. It was with mixed feelings that I found her at the hospice, as it meant that, yes, she was alive, but at the same time perhaps close to death. I wondered at the circumstances leading to her being admitted and suddenly felt appalled that I had 'abandoned' her. I was caught in an omnipotent fantasy that if I had stayed she would have been doing better, would have taken up her bed and walked. So it was with not inconsiderable anxiety and jet-lag that I drove out to see her the following day, concerned about what of her I would find remaining.

In the hospice the soles of my shoes squeaked at a reverberating and dissonant pitch as I made my way along the pristine polished corridors, sounding like a flock of storm-driven seagulls making their way towards the bed of my lost friend.

It was at once a shock and a relief to find her, as the cancer had not been patient. Her skin was grey, her limpid and listless eyes devoid of the irreverent glint. She was half sitting, half lying on the bed, eyes half closed, still and brittle like an ancient book, as if the merest wing beat might blow her to dust and all eternity. I thought of Pop, and part of me wanted to run away but, for the first time, I sat without invitation. It was extraordinary to be back there with her. I said the word that had gained such a passionate foothold in my heart: 'Val'.

The pilgrim's eyelids lifted slightly. It seemed to take a lot out of her, just doing that. 'What the hell has happened to you?' I shouted inside, but I knew, and I couldn't ask her how she was doing because she wasn't; it was being done to her. So I sat with her and I waited quietly. Her lips parted into the merest hint but unmissable trace of a smile, a smile that betrayed a mouth so full of ulcers that they had spread onto her lips and face. The tissue paper hand that lay on the bed twitched ever so slightly, so I took it in mine as gently as I could and felt hot tears well up inside me.

A visitor arrived full of reasoned intent, haemorrhaging a sort of rigorous goodwill and vigorous health all over the ward. She would have left most of us feeling depressed and anaemic in comparison, let alone a patient in a hospice ward already feeling an unsurpassable wasteland lay between them and the 'living'. The visitor had heard Val was 'poorly' so had baked a magnificent and redemptive chocolate cake. She insisted on 'at least a slice!' as she vended the life-assuring qualities of food like some snake oil salesman riding into town.

She hadn't noticed the ulcers; I don't think she really noticed Val. The smiling visitor's aggressive heartiness seemed dreadfully insensitive to me, and I struggled for something to put her off her stride. But Val whispered extremely quietly and slowly to her, 'Thank you . . . that's very kind . . . I'm talking with Paul . . . Thanks for coming.'

A wonderful moment. The woman had run aground on

Val's straight-forwardness. Stunned but still talking and smiling, the visitor retreated. Even before she had turned away, it was possible to catch the first glimpse of a smug and haughty disdain rising majestically on the visitor's face like a new sun.

I was brought back by a weak squeeze of my hand from the Val beside me, not from the Val I had left behind. 'I'm not doing so well,' she said.

'So I see, Val.'

'They're taking good care of me here,' she said as she glanced around for some evidence that this was so. But all she could come back with was, 'It's not so bad.'

'I've missed you,' I said, my voice cracking.

She nodded, tears in her eyes. 'Help me sit up a bit.'

Feeling clumsy and awkward I half lifted, half pushed her to a semi-recline, and noticed as I did so some inward rallying of spirit in her. She seemed to notice a change in her state as well, for she whispered rather quizzically, 'Tell me, Paul, what is it exactly you *do*?'

Good question. I had thought about that a great deal without having formulated anything coherent, so I had no pat answer. It was quiet in the hospice, too quiet at times, as if such unspeakable things had happened through the night that the inmates and staff were sworn to silence. The unspeakable was death. A bed near you that was occupied when you went to sleep was empty on your waking. Nothing was said. The woman in the bed opposite was staring at us, perhaps wondering if it would be she or Val next, hoping it would be Val or hoping it would be herself; it's always hard to know.

Like most of the visitors, this patient looked terminally lost, cast out and abandoned in her little boat in the dark of darkest night, a faraway lantern vaguely visible, swaying in the deep black.

'Well,' I said in a voice of quiet confidence when I hadn't a clue what mysteries were about to emanate from my mouth, 'it's like you're on this journey, Val.' She seemed to straighten in herself at these words, her eyes slightly more alive and focused. 'It's a long journey, and you've got some sense that you might be somewhere near the end of it, but you're not sure. You haven't been on this journey before so there is no way of telling. You're travelling along really slow, as if you're on a wagon or something.' I waited for the next piece to come to me. Val was as still as a monk.

It did: 'You've happened to come across me on the side of the road, and I've asked if it would be OK with you if I climbed up beside you on your wagon. You've let me get on board, and so here I am.'

And then the next part arrived, 'Sometimes you may try to give me the reins, but I won't take them, no matter how you try to get me to. You're driving, it's your wagon, and it's your journey. I tell you what I can see from up there beside you, and at times I can see things you can't, so I point them out if I think that could be helpful. I don't have to know how or why. But I never tell you what to do or where to go, and I do my best to keep out of your way.

'In the back of the wagon, there's this huge pile of shit.' Her eyebrows gave a surprised salute at this, 'You know it's there, and I know it's there, and I know that you know, and you know that I know. But you also know that you can ignore it if you want; that's up to you. But if you want to look at it, then I'll sift through it with you. I won't change the subject, and I won't say it's OK if it isn't, and I won't leave the room if you start talking about dying or cancer or if you're upset.

'As long as you want me on the wagon. I'll be there. If you ever want me to get off, then I will, no argument. It's your wagon. And if you ever want to pick me up again, that'll be OK too. It's up to you. You see, I know I'm lucky to be up here with you; I see it as a privilege. So that's what I do.'

'Yes . . .' she whispered, 'that's it. You're my compassionate companion.'

That went right into me. On my report for the day I wrote:

Val has accepted nothing more can be done for her medically. She has accepted she is dying but unsure how long it will take.

For me the main focus of the visit was reconnecting and reaffirming that, in Val's words, 'We will make the rest of the journey together.'

This is when you begin to find out just how close you have become.

'Giddyup,' said the myeloma.

THE TWO RINGS

That same week I got another call from the hospice. Would I come? I drove out of the city, past the turn-off to Val's home feeling a pang of dread in my gut, out to the building in which she would die. As I arrived at her bedside, Val slowly, quietly asked, 'Do you notice anything different?'

A wild white sparse shock of hair, spectacles hanging down on a cord and folded over her ample bosom, pink diaphanous nightshirt, wrinkled paper-skinned arms, hands folded left over right upon her lap, bedlinen neat across her body, the red *Rubaiyat* closed beside her covered legs. Her eyes were redder and more weepy than usual, her face more gaunt, her voice weaker. She had deteriorated rapidly, but I didn't think it was this development she was referring to.

Running out of patience, shorter of time than most, she said, 'My rings fell off last night.' As her words entered me, time and space curved away as Einstein predicted, a quiet cocooned us from and the rest of the world.

'Your rings . . .' I said.

She wriggled the fingers of her left hand and said, 'My wedding ring and my eternity ring.' She was speaking slowly, carefully, and with a tone of quiet conspiracy. 'They slipped off my finger. I woke with a fright and knew straight away they were missing. I wondered what on earth could have happened. I thought they'd been stolen, right off my finger. But they hadn't. Good thing too. I found them beside my pillow.' She gave a little practised frown and shook her head, 'Isn't that odd.' She raised an eyebrow at me. It took her a long time to get all of this out. She moved across her words like a fox over breaking ice.

'They're back on I see,' I said, as my head bowed involuntarily towards the numinous rings.

'Yes, but they didn't just *come off*, did they? They must have come off for a reason. To tell me something,' she said, firm. 'They weren't on the floor, where you'd expect them to be. Or in the sheets. They were right beside my pillow. I knew that meant something.'

I just nodded, and seeing me nod she looked pleased. As pleased as she could look considering her predicament. Val is the only person I have known who could smile by merely raising one eyebrow.

'Another puzzle,' she said, 'and I've been thinking about it.' She looked very serious, Life had become a very serious business for her. 'Something's changed, that's for sure. I can feel it. My Lifeline stopping, my rings coming off . . .' She nodded to herself at this and I felt how cool the space around her bed had become, even though the wards were always stifling.

'I can't remember when I would have had my wedding ring off last,' she said. 'It's never come off by itself before.' She was talking, slowly, not really to me, but talking so I could witness what she was saying. 'It wasn't worth much, Tom and I didn't have money when we got married. Once we did have a bit, he bought me this eternity ring, and so I put that on second.

'But when I saw the rings beside my pillow, I knew I had to put them on the other way around,' she said, holding up her hand. 'And that's what it means, that's the answer to this puzzle: I should put the eternity ring back on first. I need to know that . . . that I'm closer to eternity than anything else now.'

I felt my heart heave. She knew. I didn't feel sad, and she didn't seem to either. It was a strange feeling, somehow reassuring. It seemed to us that, for this to happen, Val must be known, the Gods must have remembered her, had never forgotten. And when she died, a messenger would be sent out over the universe, as in an old Bushmen story, to inform all creation that someone who was once upright, had now fallen.

Val was beginning to live some kind of unity now. We could feel it. Nothing needed to be said about it directly. We had got there – not needing to spell things out – by breaking the pond and dispersing the pile of magazines and all the essential things that happened and were done and were left behind. Without these things, we could never really have *begun* to talk. She was repairing some tap-root in her that had been cut. Drowning, surrender, re-connection. Val's fingers were skeletal, and the rings were very loose, but they didn't come off again until they were removed, and given to Christine.

RUTTERS AND HYDROGRAPHERS
22 February 1995

Sent for again, *veni, vedi*. After I sat down in the straight-backed chair by Val's metal bed, she whispered, 'What have you seen me go through?'

To get this much out was an effort for her. 'In general terms, do you mean?'

'Mmm. The steps.'

'Well, there is a model I know, but it won't entirely fit because it's only a map; it can't be the terrain itself, not the real thing. But I can tell you that, if you want.' Val slowly pointed to a pad of paper and a pen at the side of her bed. I hadn't been expecting this from Val, yet I felt completely ready. I picked up the paper and pen. She'd been preparing for this question, obviously. 'Write,' she said. I wasn't too sure about doing this. If Val wanted a map that was going to be of any use to her, then she'd have to carry on charting it herself. In nautical terms, centuries ago such a book would be called a *rutter*. A rutter was a sort of guidebook, left by a ship's master or hydrographer who had navigated uncharted waters. The rutter was written when sailing in new seas, like Val was in dying, and as I was doing with Val, and in my own life. But there was no rutter that could take into account the changing forces of Nature – the tides or changing currents or storms or doldrums or heat or cold. So that's what mastery means – not that you don't go off course or get lost or screw things up badly at times. Mastery is when you can see when you are off course, and you set a new course, and navigate your way through it. And all along experience tells you you will be swept off course again.

But Val wanted a map. So I put the pad on the bed beside her, where she could easily read it. There was a general map, from Elisabeth Kübler-Ross's book *On Death and Dying*. For want of anything better, I decided to lay it out for Val. I wrote on the pad back to front and upside down, a skill I'd picked up in my years in business. I could read whatever documents the person on the other side of the desk had in front of him. Somehow this intruding knack had translated into the ability to write this way as well. I wrote

DENIAL

'The first place you'd usually go after the shock of diagnosis, after the shock of being told something like, "We're very sorry to have to tell you this, but you have cancer,"' I said, but stopped dead when I saw Val's eyes harden. I wondered whether she was remembering being given The News? Tom had been there beside her, supposedly as fit as a fiddle.

'This model isn't like a straight line, Val. You can go back and forth through the stages, up and down the steps, even be on different steps at the same time. But it gives some sort of vague outline to what can happen.' I'd known all this stuff before I'd met Val, and it didn't help me very much. The true rutter would begin and end with this: anything can happen, in any way, to anybody, at any time, in any place, with any outcome, and it was always destined to happen that way. Val raised her left hand from the bed, a forefinger just pushed forward and out, enough for it to be a point and make the point that I was to get on with it.

'The news can be just too much for someone to take in, so they don't. They can't face it. So they sort of deny it, and maybe hope it'll just go away.' I stopped there.

Inch by inch her head moved, side to side. She was insulted that I could even *think* she'd ever experienced such a place. 'Nope,' she said, so I let that one go.

ISOLATION

'Part of denial is called isolation,' I said, 'which is where you sort of split into two people, like you have a twin. It's like one of you knows you're really sick or dying, and can talk about it; while the other part of you seems to know nothing about it.' Val's head moved again.

She didn't like this much. 'Nothing to do with me,' she said, not to give an example of what I'd just been talking about, but because she was irritated I could imply such a thing about her. She pointed again to the paper.

Feeling a bit wary, I wrote

ANGER

on the little pad. Val's eyes bulged.

This didn't seem to be going so well, and I said, 'Maybe this isn't very helpful, Val.'

Quietly, firmly, she said, 'Keep going. Why anger? We all know we're going to die.'

'I don't think we all do, Val, not really *know* it. Otherwise we wouldn't live like we do. We wouldn't find petty things so vital. We live as if we'll somehow be magically ready to die when the time comes, as if we don't have to prepare for it at all. We think we'll be better off if we don't think about . . .' I caught myself on my hobby-horse. I shut-up. Val looked at me as if I was trying to sell her heroin. Then she gave herself a little nod, and went straight to sleep.

What on earth was I doing? While I waited, I wrote in my diary and breathed in syncopation with her. This last had become my habit. It helped me tune in to what was going on inside her, and seemed to close the gap between us. It was the first time her outward breaths were longer than her inward ones. I wondered if it was going to be anything like this when she died. I wondered about that a great deal.

'Anger.' Val had woken back into her thoughts as if she hadn't been away.

'Yes,' I said. 'You realise this thing *is* happening to you, and has been dumped on you without you having any choice about it. Even though there've been billions of precedents, you're angry because you're not in control of . . .'

'No,' Val cut in, 'never angry,' and she tapped the paper with her finger. Angrily.

'OK.' I was pontificating again. I wrote

BARGAINING

Val looked across at me as if I was some sort of lunatic, driving with one wheel in the sand, but I would keep going unless she told me to stop.

'Bargaining is where you think, "If I do this or that, I'll get better." You might think, "As long as I eat something every day then I'll stay alive." And so you do that, you eat even if you don't want any food or it's really horrendous to eat anything. You eat because food becomes life. That's the deal. Or you might think, "If I go to church and repent, then God will take this punishment, this illness that is my penance, God will take it away. And then I'll be OK." Something like that. So that's bargaining, and sometimes friends and family get right into it as well, trying to get you to eat or see the vicar or something.' Val had begun to shake her head again, so I tried a new thread.

'Another way you might bargain is by setting some date in the future, some date that will be the end. Like an anniversary or something.' I stopped there because Val was still shaking her head. She pointed back to the piece of paper on the side of the bed.

I took a breath, then wrote

DEPRESSION

'This, if it all went in a straight line, which as I said it doesn't, is the fourth stage,' I said.

'Depression?' she said, glaring. '*Depression?*'

'Yes, Val, depression.'

'I suppose you'd better tell me,' she conceded, not impressed at all.

'When the bargaining doesn't work, and you realise you really are very sick and that you might not get better, then that can really knock you for six. You can feel just about everything a person is capable of feeling, but with an intensity you might not have experienced before. So it's not only that you suffer, it's that you have this constant *awareness* that you are suffering and are going to suffer. Like drowning, and all the time knowing you're drowning.' That one caught me by surprise. Where had *that* come from?

'But what are you going to do, when most people around you are so embarrassed by your situation? When most people really do not want to know. So who can you offload onto, when you know and no one else seems to know?' I paused, Val was thinking about this one.

When she glanced back at me, I said, 'Then there is the loss. It's like an endless outgoing tide. It continuously tugs away at everything you think is your self and your life. I reckon depression is quite a healthy response to all this.'

Deep in thought for a while, she eventually shook her head

and said, 'Haven't heard anything I like yet. Sure you've got this right?' Responses began rushing through my head, but I sat there, and I waited. She pointed at the piece of paper, and I wrote

∀CCEPT∀NCE

Her eyes moved from the word to the far wall. She fixed on some point in the middle distance, alert like a mouse at the crack of an open door.

'You might jump about a bit,' I said, 'or experience nothing of what I've just said at all. But if you go *through* the depression and not away from it, you might come to something approaching acceptance.' At last, a nod from that exasperating old head. I think a lot of the time that's how we found each other – exasperating. The Chinese say: Where there is always harmony in the home, there is no love.

'Acceptance isn't like everything is suddenly OK; it's more that the struggle has pretty much ended. You'll still be hanging out for a cure, a reprieve, because hope seems to remain, no matter what. But you can accept where you are, and you've come to terms with it. So this can be a more peaceful and meaningful time, where things aren't so tense and anxious.'

'Yes,' Val said. 'At last you've said something that makes some sense.' Her body relaxed in this new and hard won place. 'Acceptance. That's where I am.' She looked up at me, 'Thank you, Paul.' She said it very tenderly. You don't have to say much.

Her old hand crept out for the piece of paper, and I handed it to her. She rolled her fingers at me to motion for the pen, so I gave her that too. Then she began to twist around to reach her *Rubaiyat*, so I got up and put it on her lap. We had come naturally to this place where she didn't have to ask, and was happy for me to do these little things for her. On the old red well-read book, she supported the little inaccurate map of the last part of her life. And with pen pressed hard into the paper, she crossed off shakily, one by one, the words I had written upside down on the page. But she left unmarked, there on the bottom of that little piece of paper

ACCEPTANCE

Trembling fingers slowly folded the map, until only the final word was visible. She gave herself a little nod, and immediately fell asleep. It seemed such a deep sleep, I knew there would be no more talking with her that day. So I sat with her for twenty minutes or so, breathing with her. I thought a little about what had just happened, wondering where she was now, and if she would come back. As usual, Val had the last word.

BENEATH THE BOUGH
28 February 1995

It was a few days before Val's seventy-sixth birthday, and I was there at the hospice sharing a sickly sweet sherry with her. She rummaged through her *Rubaiyat*.

> *Here with a Loaf of Bread beneath the Bough,*
> *A Flask of Wine, a Book of Verse – and Thou*
> *Beside me singing in the Wilderness –*
> *And Wilderness is Paradise enow.*

I found myself so profoundly moved and reconstituted on being with her that I began to recognise the difficulties that lay ahead for myself as she moved inexorably towards death. I felt flutterings of a fleeting concern that this old woman whom I loved might be better off and more at ease were I just to let her get on with it by herself. But more persistent was an inexplicable sureness in me that the Gods wanted more from Val and more from our relationship. Regardless of what unfolded within and without me, it was Val who was clear that I was to continue my visits 'until the end'.

She was disillusioned and disappointed, weak and

chronically ill, and had reluctantly forfeited almost all vestiges of choice and control. Yet within this decay lay seeds of wisdom and redemption. Over the weeks that followed, Val began to talk less about her cancer, although its presence was by no means forgotten. It ate away at her corporeally and psychically, always somewhere not far enough away, a Gollum scratching and slithering in the back of her mind, through the marrow of her bones.

I visited Val as often as I could. I turned up one afternoon, expected and anally on time, to find her asleep in her hospice bed. I sat down beside her and waited. When she eventually woke she was in the frame of mind and full of enough vitality for a chat about anything insubstantial, and so it was for four hours. I wrote in my notes that she was 'confused about her prognosis', which meant she was wondering if she would be 'released' from the hospice. She said 'released' now more out of a feeling that it *should* be what she wanted, rather than because it was. And indeed she was at large the following week, 'for a day at home!' One last look at the life she was leaving, a review of the ship before she was scuppered and sunk.

It was a cold blank day as we pulled up outside the house under an oppressive steel sky. The house was frigid, destitute. Going inside was like entering a tomb, with vapour coming out of our mouths. Val scanned for some connection to what had once been everything to her, all that she would have fought for, all that she and Tom had made out of this world. I could see in the set of her shoulders, the sinking forward of her head, the turning this way and that, that there was nothing there for her now.

Exhausted by the short journey to the house, Val sat not on the sofa but on one of the matching armchairs. It was pointed directly at the television set and probably aligned, just so, for decades. Val looked forlorn. She was not going to have the wrenching farewell to all she was losing, the tug that would have confirmed the value of her life. Instead she had to experience the total lack of relevance of what had been all, but had at the last shown itself, in shame, to be utterly insignificant. We remained silent, as befitted the atmosphere of mourning. Val's position could not have been clearer: she was not interested in this place, it meant nothing to her. It was as though on her final parole into the world she had chosen to spend her time at McDonald's. Her disappointment was palpable. She sat in the chair staring at her distorted reflection in the television screen where she had spent so long in search of consolation and connection.

On the way over in the car she had been telling me, in a long, slow exhausted sort of way, how much pressure she was feeling to be 'cheery' with people. She felt obliged to be upbeat for others no matter what she was actually feeling. She told me people were encouraging this display, ostensibly for her benefit rather than their own. She felt there was little opportunity for her to be miserable, to grieve. Now she was having time. Now she had no choice.

We stayed in that room for hours, with nothing to be said that was not already being so austerely spoken by the barren house. At least she wasn't alone. I wondered how many, how many billions would die in my lifetime with no-one else really there with them. It was cold there, but we lit no fires and turned on no heaters. We just sat there in our coats, becalmed in stagnant waters.

PRECIPICE
Thursday 16 March 1995

There was a fire in Val's eyes when I arrived at her bedside. Once I was seated, she said, 'I've been waiting for you to come.' She looked both excited and depleted. 'I knew I couldn't tell anyone else; they wouldn't be able to understand. So I had to wait for you.' There was a muted tone of admonition, as if warning me I should always come when called for. I was to fail her on this count.

Sitting on the uncomfortable chair, squeezed between the wall and her bed, I waited as Val drew breath and sorted out her thoughts. 'I've had a dream, a magnificent dream,' she said.

'Ah.' I was pleased. So a dream had come. I had been hoping she would tell me her dreams.

'Except it wasn't a dream,' she added.

She took some time to get her breathing together again. She could sense my curiosity, and obviously wanted to draw this out. 'It wasn't a dream,' she said again. 'I went to another level of consciousness.' She gave herself that affirming little nod of the head. 'I knew it wasn't a dream,' she said, 'because all the time I knew I was there, and not here, if you see what I mean.'

I nodded, 'Mmm, I believe I do.'

'It was night,' she said, 'and I knew I should have been here in my bed and that I wasn't. I was somewhere else and something remarkable happened there.' Val adjusted the sleeves of her garishly pink and disturbingly see-through nightgown, patted her re-establishing hair, and then turned and gave me a cheeky smile, a cocky raise of an eyebrow. I felt I was soon to be let into a great secret, as if I was back in my childhood with a friend who was about to divulge some shocking account of what the grown-ups do.

Looking into and through me, gazing far beyond the bounds of the hospice ward, out beyond the town and the world, she said, 'I was on a horse.' She paused there, stirrup engaged, as if to remount.

'It was a beautiful huge white horse, and I was riding it. I don't think I can ride but I could there. I was riding this huge horse, and we were galloping towards the edge of a precipice. We were going very very fast. I don't think I've ever felt anything like it. I was really frightened and I suddenly realised, "This horse is going to run right off the edge!" and I didn't want it to, because somehow I knew that it was a long long way down, and that would be It. So I thought that I must stop the horse and it stopped right away, as soon as I thought it.'

She looked pleased about this, smiled three teeth and shrugged. People were going about their business on the ward: the woman in the opposite bed, in some other world, stared over myopically; a woman looked around in fear and trembling as she rolled a steel trolley of tea and biscuits menacingly amongst the steel beds; a family gathered around a patient but looked only at shoes or through the window; a young man tried to listen to an old dying woman.

'Once we had stopped, I didn't feel quite so frightened any more, and I thought to myself, "While I'm here, I might as well have a bit of a look around." So I did! I got down from the horse, and it wasn't so bad really. I realised that I actually quite liked it there, and I began to have a look. I was drawn to the edge of the precipice and went over to it. I was amazed,' she said with a raise of eyebrows. 'I just couldn't believe my eyes.

'There, way way down, and stretching as far as I could see, in all directions, was a city of light. Everything there was made of light. Everything! And I just stood there and stared at it. I don't know how long I stood there; it might have been all night, but I just couldn't take my eyes off it. It was so beautiful. I'd never thought I would see anything like that.'

She paused there for a while, on the edge, admiring the view, and this time I waited there with her. 'Then I heard a voice,' she said, and turned to look at me. 'And the voice told me to give *you* two messages.' She stopped there, on the edge. It was an amazing moment. I had been thrashing about, struggling for oxygen in my life, while way over my head there had always been an infinity of air. And now, all of a sudden, here I was back on the surface, being given a breath, two breaths. This was not what I had expected to happen next in my life.

'I was told it was very important I pass the messages on

to you,' she said, and a chill ran through me in the warm hospice room.

'That's why I've been waiting for you to come,' she said. 'I remember them, word for word, because I've heard them before.'

My heart was in my mouth, and I started to feel incredibly full throughout my body, as if there would be no room in me at all for whatever she was about to say.

Val stared at me, waiting. 'So, do you want to hear them or not?'

'Yes, I do,' I said, vaguely nodding at her. 'This isn't what I was expecting at all.'

With a syncopated patting down of the sheets on each side of her legs, well in control of the situation, she said, 'Right, this is what I was asked to tell you. The first thing comes from *Hamlet*: "This above all: to thine own self be true, / And it must follow, as the night the day, / Thou canst not then be false to any man." There.' A definite nod of her head. 'What do you think of that then?'

I wasn't quite sure whether she was asking about the message or her ability to recite it. I was quieted. I knew the piece, and I had always been deeply impressed by it. And now here it was, arriving in my lap as Fate, as I sat by the bed of a dying woman. I said nothing, and I looked down into my hands thinking how far away I was from the place Polonius advised.

It was as if God had suddenly turned up in the ward, and told me He'd had me on His mind for a while, and that this was what He thought. I'd not been forgotten. It was I who had turned away. But there was more, and Val was short of time, as short as you and I. She said, 'And then I was told to tell you this, and I know this one too because it comes from the *Rubaiyat*, and Tom gave me that book years ago. The stanza goes: "The Moving Finger writes; and, having writ, / Moves on: nor all their Piety nor Wit / Shall lure it back and cancel half a Line, / Nor all your Tears wash out a Word of it."'

'Jesus.' I shook my head and looked up at the ceiling. 'Christ.' It's a joy to be hidden, but a tragedy not to be found.

I was flooded by great benevolent forces. Not forgotten. And I knew then that Val, the *Angelo*, the messenger, my Hermes Trismegistus, was very close to death.

KNOTS
Sunday 19 March 1995

The phone rang late on a Sunday afternoon. It was the hospice passing on a message from Val – would I visit her, now? I was tired from weeks of work without a day off: seeing patients, running the hospice training, supervising psychotherapy students, facilitating training weekends. It was a good 90-minute drive from home to the hospice, on the sort of cold night that you really want to spend at home.

'Tell Val I'll be there as soon as I can,' I said. It wasn't saintliness; it was that I wanted to be with Val more than I needed to rest. It was already dark by the time I left home, with an uneasiness in my stomach as the old car deafeningly ground out the miles along the soulless grey motorways. The little VW seemed at odds with being a car at all, and definitely at odds with being out on such a dreadful night.

I parked under the mad waving trees outside the main hospice building. Trees seem to me nocturnal creatures, displaying the beauty and passivity of sleeping children during the day, and coming menacingly alive and full of possibility when darkness falls. The hospice itself was a squat brick building, uninviting, shut up on a wet and windy night with its temporary passengers. A port in a storm, only one-way tickets for sale, no first class, no baggage, no timetable, no known destination, too much waiting, then suddenly: gone.

I walked across the windswept driveway of the hospice with half an eye on the flailing maelstrom above me. The front doors, glass, yellow light spilling out onto the steps. This was the line, the frontier. This is where we hesitated, us visitors, if not outwardly then inwardly, as we stood on the threshold that separated the dying from the world. This was where we were no longer sure. This was where it became so much harder to pretend we were. The reception area, functional and empty; still time to retreat, to flee, without being noticed. On into the shining hallway, hearts in our mouths, breathing getting a little more difficult.

The bright lights struck out unsympathetically, violently, at the visitors. I passed them by and squeaked down the polished floors of the corridors, turned right – big squeak – and walked in to find Val upright in her tidy anodyne bed, surrounded by duplicitous antibacterial whiteness.

She beamed at me, a gentle three-toothed wizened beam, and with her left hand slowly pointed to the chair, just for me. I sat, still, quiet. A thought of the draining return journey came into my mind but, as the Buddhists would say, it was not invited to tea. Then another thought appeared. I wondered whether I had been playing God with Val, nudging and prodding her towards the sort of death I wanted her to have. And when she had stepped outside the area that was safe for her, outside where she had wanted to go, did I push her?

Reaching under her blanket, Val took out a knotted bloom of pink yarn about the size of a cricket ball. She held it up, head height, and looked at me to make sure I had noticed it. I looked at the wool. I looked back at Val. She looked like death; she looked full of wonder.

Forensically she probed with her thin fingers and her whole being deep into the wool. It took a while before her fingers emerged, producing an end, a beginning to the strand. She held it up in a shaking hand, head height. She looked at me again, and I looked again at the wool and again back at her, to see a slight raising of an eyebrow.

She gently, patiently kneaded the strand out of the knots, rolled what she had onto two fingers, and held this up for me to see. I went through my routine: Val – wool – Val, except it was not a routine, it was becoming more and more a ritual of a natural and profound order. I was altar boy to her high priest. She saw that I saw, she understood that I understood, each was affected by how the other was affected. Val went back to her searching and unknotting, respectfully, thoroughly, tolerantly. I took it all in, as much as I could. I looked compassionately and diligently on what she showed me at each point along the way. And I quietly waited as it all unfolded, completely out of my hands.

Each time she extracted a further length of thread, she rolled it up, looked at it, held it in the air for me to see, to recognise, to remember. She then returned to the entrails for more of the strand. I was totally engrossed, a part of the unfolding pattern.

After no more than an hour, or two, the knots and mess and tangle were undone. Val triumphantly raised the ball of wool aloft, disentangled. She turned her old head to mine, tears in her eyes, lips trembling, and nodded, almost bowed to me. She said with great difficulty and gentleness, 'Thank you so much for coming, Paul.' She was thanking me for everything. For thinking about her when I was on the bus or in New Zealand; for ringing around to find her; for carrying the biscuits from the kitchen; for not telling her I had *my* Gods; for being equally at home talking about re-incarnation and the shape of tea bags; for stifling my yawns; for screwing the leg back on the arm-chair, for not crying or hugging her even if *I* wanted to.

'Thanks for having me along, Val.'

And then, she lay her head back on the large accommo-dating pillows, and fell instantly asleep. Her hair pushed out, white on the warm white.

By the time I hit the cold air of the evening, everything in the world had slowed down. I sat in my little car, waiting for it to warm up. I rarely did this, but I realised I cared about that car, that extraordinary, brilliant, little car. I looked up at the night sky, overawed by the moon and the clouds. It wasn't just the moon or the clouds, it was The Moon and The Clouds. I was intensely encountering what it was to be alive. And It was almost more than I could bear. It was all just too extra-ordinary. I looked at the trees, and they looked as though their roots went all the way to the centre of the earth.

I understood that Val was far more alive than I was, than I had ever been, more alive than anyone I knew. And as I wended my way by highway and byway back to London, it occurred to me that when Val had lain back and fallen asleep, she may have died at that very moment. It would have been more than enough time.

WORDS FIND
Wednesday 22 March 1995

Val's face contorted as if she were chewing on a small live animal. She managed to spit out a 'Word'. My heart sank while she chewed some more, as if searching for something between her teeth.

'Find' found a way to escape her mouth. It took her about a minute to get that much out. And it wasn't *that* exactly, it was more 'w w w fi fie were nd were . . .'

> *'Is there anybody there?' said the Traveller,*
> *Knocking on the moonlit door . . .*

I put 'word' and 'find' together, then she said 'Together'. Her mind was in one hell of a mess, and it was difficult enough experiencing her problem from the outside, the very outside. She was telling me that all of the words were in there, together in her mind, but she couldn't get them to come out in the right order.

I had arrived to find that Val had suffered a stroke. It had left her, as the nurse in sublime understatement said, 'somewhat incapacitated'. I was left to discover for myself exactly what this meant, and I discovered we were losing a route to each other. Everything would be taken.

So I said, 'The words are there in your head, Val, but you just can't manage to get them out in the same way that they're in there. Is it something like that?'

She nodded, sighed with relief, and after a great deal of struggle managed, 'Minor'.

'Yes, they told me as I came in, Val. They told me you've had a minor stroke and they weren't sure what the effects of it had been. One of them is that you can't get your words out, which must be very frustrating,' I said.

She nodded.

> 'Tell them I came, and no one answered,
> That I kept my word,' he said . . .

'When you've had enough energy and I've been here you've always used it to talk. Now it's almost impossible to even do that. You're probably wondering how many more chances you're going to have to talk. Is it something like that, Val?'

Her head gave that one little nod.

'Feel free to have a go, Val,' I said. 'I'll wait while you do what you can do.'

It was excruciating for her and it lasted for hours. She managed to tell me, with me doing much of the filling in, that losing her mind had always frightened her. That and physical pain were her two great dreads. She had talked about this before, but now there was no separation of the subject from the subject. Although she could think, she could not talk, and that was leaving her cut-off and terrified.

'Can you write?'

She held up a trembling hand. She could barely raise it. What she feared most, now she could not talk, was something happening to her and not being able to tell anyone about it or ask for help. She had lost her main link to others, her only resource for protecting herself from whatever was to come.

We were in the usual little ward, where privacy was in short supply. Patients in other beds could easily listen in, even join in. And some tried. Visitors often considered it their duty to greet one and all with their lively abundance, mixed with a practised solemnity. Val's was the first bed they would come across, and so she was commonly subjected to the strangers' opening salvo. Nurses came and went, with trolley and medication and doctor and tea and magazine and all sorts of business equally superfluous but gratefully distracting to many a patient and visitor alike. There could be a patient in the bed opposite in complete despair, or 'entertaining' a terrified visiting family, or staring open-mouthed and dribbling and without blinking, to the point where I would wonder if they had already expired. And this, all of this, constituted the arena for our meeting: Val's new lounge.

Out of her misfiring mind, Val brought up her aunt. She had been recently featuring in our conversations, because Val had scheduled she would not die until her aunt had 'passed on'. Her aunt was in a 'retirement' home, and while she lived Val would live, and so it must be.

Why Val would make such an effort to speak about this, of all things, suddenly became clear to me and struck me as

awful: she was no longer eager that her aunt should live, and
so stave off Val's death; she was concerned *about* her aunt
continuing to live, and thus forcing Val to endure the hell of
living without her faculties.

I left Val that afternoon, both of us badly shaken.

And how the silence surged softly backward,
When the plunging hooves were gone.

THE SILENT POND
Friday 24 March 1995

Two days later I arrived back at the hospice in my usual position: wondering what on earth I would find, and feeling a mixture of excitement, sadness and uncertainty. A nurse told me Val was 'feeling much better in herself, now she can put her words together again'.

'I've been waiting to tell you about it,' Val said, labouring out every word. There was a hand-written sticker with 'Val Hall' in black marker pen stuck on the bedframe beside her head. Perhaps there were new staff around. Perhaps people were having trouble recognising her. Perhaps she was a product on a shelf, returned, unwanted.

'I've been to another level of consciousness again,' she said. I felt a chill run through me, shiver from my gut up my spine to the back of my head, then down my torso, cool into my stomach. I was visiting Val as much as I could, but getting more and more exhausted. I was overloaded and it was entirely my fault, but her words immediately reanimated me.

'So . . .' I said.

'I was there, on a bridge,' she said, gazing out. 'I was standing right over the Silent Pond.' I felt the same chill again, and knew Val had been on the edge of death. Her every word entered every pore of my skin, like millions of tiny acupuncture needles.

'I was just standing there looking down into the Silent Pond,' she said, and stopped, to look again. The deep darkness of it reflected in her watery pupils. 'It was ever so dark, endlessly dark. I couldn't see into it at all. But I knew it was eternally deep. It went down and down and never stopped. It was quite something to be standing over it, on this old, old bridge that had been there forever.'

Everything had gone totally quiet inside and outside of me. There was only Val's voice and the eternally deepening silence.

'And then I realised something. I realised that if I crossed the bridge, if I went right over to the other side, then I would never come back. And then,' she said, 'do you know what?'

'What?'

With a shrug of her pink taffeta shoulders, she said, 'I remembered what we were having for breakfast, so I decided to come back.'

FACE
Saturday 25 March – day

I would sit beside Val as she lay back against her pillows, her head at the level of my heart. She said little since she tired easily and seemed to flit in and out of life itself. Sometimes in mid-sentence she would leave, only to continue that same sentence two or twenty minutes later. I would sit there, no longer waiting, no longer thinking, but just sitting there, listening, being with her. Before long she would return, sometimes asking if she had 'drifted off'.

'Just for a while,' I'd say, and she would look a little disgusted with herself. 'I'm not here for you to entertain me, Val.'

'Maybe,' she would force out, 'but I'm not much of a host, am I?'

No, she was not. Death was the host, and living was the invitation Val had not refused. Death threw the party and I had my invitation too. I would not be overlooked or forgotten, not then, not even if I wanted to be, nor the hospice nurses, and the doctors and the cooks and the cleaners and receptionists, the people who lived around the hospice and the people who knew them and the people who knew those people and the people who built the hospice, and the people who manufactured the things the hospice was built out of, and the people who gathered the materials together to make those things, and the people who owned or lived around the land those materials were gathered from. And you. We have all accepted the invitation to our deaths by being born; none can refuse.

'Oh, I've been asleep?' she said, but not as fast as you can read it. All had become slow motion, and enormous exertion. Any word dropped or misplaced would mean the whole sentence massive would have to be assailed once more.

'When I look in the mirror . . . my face . . .' and she fell asleep again. I sat there looking into her face as she slept. It was a radiant face. After a while I opened my diary and read some notes I'd scribbled as I sat beside her as she slept during earlier visits. One entry read:

Life is a sea of change. I, like all others, can only become frustrated when I attempt to put foundations down into that sea. I can make my boat stable, but not the sea. To stabilise the sea would be to end the ebb and flow of Life. I would be dead in my security, in my safety.

To be alive, on the other hand, is to feel the lack of safety inherent in being alive, and to go on choosing to be alive. It's about learning to sail, about choosing risk and balance . . . It's to ride with the sea and, at times, to capsise. But there's no shame in that, because the risk taken cannot be doubted. You get back in your boat, maybe make it a little more stable from what you've learned, and sail on. There is no shame in learning . . .

Only if I attempt to block the flow of Life will I be able to predict the result – Life will try to wake me up and may overwhelm me in the process . . .

'What was I saying?'

I answered after a long pause, a pause that allowed Val to prepare for the effort of gathering-in my response: 'You were talking about looking in the mirror, Val.' Timing.

'Yes,' she said, 'my face. Know what?'

Wait. I replied with a small shake of my head.

'Getting a halo. I look in the mirror, I see light. Peculiar. You notice?' She said this a little shyly. It had always been important to Val that I saw.

'I was just thinking more or less the same thing, Val. What do you make of it?'

She turned her head slowly towards me, to look me in the eye, 'I will die soon,' she said. She knew. 'You?'

'Same thing,' I said, 'that you're going to die soon, Val.' That was pretty much the whole visit. And it lasted a couple of hours. I cannot begin to explain the sense of peace, or how that peace washed through me, soaked me to the marrow. The killing in her bones was helping to regenerate me. Gratitude, I was awash with gratitude. I couldn't imagine anyone being in a more fortunate position than I, who had had the chance to be with Val in her final years.

Val's aunt had died that day. Val knew. Her path had been cleared. This left her, on the one hand, relieved that things

had turned out as she had hoped but, on the other, at the
end of the yardstick she had set on her life. She had no difficulty in coming up with another one though. But she didn't
tell me about it; I figured it out just before she died.

NO
Saturday 25 March – night

Within the magnitude and the intimacy of the silences and the space that Val and I occupied when we were together, it was still possible for me to turn away. Maureen, a loyal friend of Val's, phoned to ask if I was going to visit Val the following evening. Dog-tired from not having had a day off in three weeks, I asked, 'Is it urgent?'

'No, Val's fine,' Maureen said. 'I just popped in to see her myself. She said she just fancies another visitor tomorrow. I can't make it, and I know she'd really like to see you.'

'And how was she?' I said. I'd seen Val only hours before, but there had been more than enough time for things to have changed, radically changed.

'She's fine, really, in quite good spirits,' Maureen said. 'I just have to be going and so she asked if I could ring you.'

'Oh, so you're still with her then?'

'Yes, I'm leaving shortly.'

'OK,' I said, and then I did it: 'Can you tell Val that I won't be able to come out tomorrow night, and that I'll come and see her on Wednesday?' Wednesday was four days away. So much can change in a few seconds. It didn't sit right in my body to say I wouldn't go. I ignored what my body was telling me.

Maureen sounded disappointed when she said she would
pass my message on to Val. But it was nothing like the disappointment I felt in myself at that moment. I had been told
that Val spoke about me often and with great pride, yet I'd
been hoping the hospice wouldn't ring again for a day at
least. I needed an evening off, I wanted to rest with a clear
conscience. But I got the former at the cost of the latter.

I didn't go, and I have to live with that. There is nothing
I can do now to put it right. There was and remains this one
exception, this one time when I didn't go to Val when she
called for me. I spent hundreds of hours with her, but there
was this one night, this one decision. It was a chance to be
with her before, in the end, she wouldn't have me back.

THE LETTER
Received Tuesday 28 March 1995

23rd March: '95

My dearest Paul,

Just a line to thank you for all your kindnesses to me and I have enjoyed knowing you. Everything went off very smooth today and everyone was very helpful. I feel strangely calm and I don't think I have too long a remainder of a journey to go – it is as if I'm drifting in the Bermuda Triangle and I am 99% certain that our theories are correct. I seem to be in a silent world of my own – no hearing aid or any other distractions, or of course I can put it down to over-tiredness as I'm not used to using so much energy.

But I can't quite cut the tie – I wonder why? Another problem to solve? Or am I just putting obstacles in the way? I'll let you know tomorrow – Goodnight Paul and God Bless You. (Interval) – (25th/3/95) Well I'm still here, well at least I think I am but I seem to be flitting in and out of consciousness. I am waiting for Maureen to come and will ask her to give you a ring to see if you are free tomorrow evening to visit me for a short while.

Once again God Bless You

Love
Val

THE RUBAIYAT OF VAL AND TOM

Wednesday 29 March 1995

The letter had arrived on Tuesday 28 March. It was to be the only letter Val sent me, and had been written and posted before I turned down her request for a visit. I had become extremely busy, which in Japanese script is written with the characters *heart* and *killing*.

'Why didn't you come?' she said.

'Work, Val. I'd too much work on.' To this day I couldn't tell you why I said that; why I didn't tell her I hadn't had a break for 21 days; why I implied that she was nothing more to me than another piece of work. For me, being with Val was being immersed in Life, awash with it, tumbled over and turned inside out by Nature.

Val was having difficulty hearing because she had stopped using her hearing aid. Listening to people impinged too much on her life now. But it wasn't a lack of hearing aid this time, she just could not believe her ears. 'What?'

The disappointment between us was palpable. We both knew I had let her down badly, I had always come before. There was a short pause, only three or four minutes. We were both feeling bad. We both knew how much we cared about each other by how dire this rift felt.

To close the gap, to keep going, that is how you might get really close, and that is where you are willing to risk getting really hurt. Val had no time for gaps or judgements, so quickly things began to thaw and ease. We could both feel that as well. There was nothing Val could hang onto now, neither resentment nor disappointment. And I was learning how rapidly things can move, when you're travelling so very slowly. I was unable to hold on to an experience with Val for long, before the next one overtook it.

My saying no had only shown us how close we had become. We just needed a few minutes of quiet together to re-establish ourselves, and then Val said, 'It's time for us to say goodbye, Paul.'

It might be hard to appreciate the intimacy and love and gratitude she conveyed in those words. If I had been at her side every moment of the last months, she still would have said exactly these words at precisely this time. That's how I see it. Fate. It was always going to be this way. At the same time, this was not what I had expected to happen next.

'What the hell do you mean it's time to say goodbye, Val? We're in this together, to the *end*, remember!? You *said* so! WE. HAD. A. *DEAL*!' That's what I thought, but I didn't say a word. I just nodded. Through the tears welling in my eyes I could see the tears well in hers, then fall to dwell in the creases of her cheeks. She reached out and held my hand, and her hand was deadly cool.

I then realised the terrible thing that had been there all along, the weakness in my position. I realised I had been banking on being with Val when she died, that this was something I had wanted for myself as much as, if not more than, for her. Yet I had the chance to put that right, belatedly, immediately, to turn away from myself and towards Val, to finally love her.

'You might want me with you, Val, so you don't feel alone,' I thought, but didn't say it.

'I think I will die in two days' time,' she said. A gathering of strength for the next words, 'I need to make the last part of the journey on my own.'

I nodded. I understood. She was in a much healthier place than I was. Val was almost dead, but that was where she was meant to be. I was almost dead as well, and that was what I was learning.

'Sometimes I wonder if I have let you down, Paul,' she said, very quietly. 'I couldn't be as strong as you wanted me to be.' This was exactly what I did not want to hear, that I was still bringing my needs to the table, well hidden under a cloak of self-righteous benevolence. To realise this, and accept it, and not to just push it away, was not easy.

'There wasn't anything you had to do for me, Val.' But as I said it, I knew I couldn't quite believe it. Val had done so much for me, still was doing. And perhaps she had to, perhaps it was her fate, as much as it was mine to be her companion. We sat there for five, maybe ten minutes, quiet. I began to relax again, let go, breathe with her. Val tenderly nursing me through this last place; it was entirely the opposite of what I had expected. All this time our eyes lay tearfully on each other's.

'I don't know how to thank you,' she said.

Hot tears welled again in my eyes, 'And I don't know how to thank you.' The gratitude between us was immense. She was happy I had made it, many years late, but I had made it now.

Another long silence ensued, the penultimate hush. Her *Rubaiyat* lay loyally on the bed beside her, festooned with strips of torn paper marking favoured stanzas. Val tapped gently on its fading red cover and said, 'I want you to have this, Paul, so you'll always remember me,' and all I could do was stare into her eyes.

'Open the cover,' she said.

I looked away to pick up the red book, and I felt as if I was leaving her. This was to be part of the leaving, the rest had already been done. It had been done as well as we could manage, with our damage and our weakness and our hope. I opened the book, and written on the back of the first page was

'That's all I could manage to write,' Val said. 'I thought you'd better have a go.' So I picked up the pen, and she dictated to me, once again, the lines of Shakespeare from her dream. But when it came to 'canst not then be false', I wrote 'canst be false'. I thought 'canst' meant 'can't', and that Val was getting the quote wrong. I thought I knew better than her. Even then. She carefully watched what I had written – of course – and her eyes widened in surprise. She looked up at me: editor of Shakespeare, editor of Val. And I, *it must follow as night follows the day*, continued confusing what was false with what was true. But she didn't say anything about it, she just let that one go, and got on with what she was doing.

To Paul, -
   This above all to thine own self be true
   and then it must surely follow as night
   must day, thou canst be false to any man.

She motioned for the pen and the book, a flick of her fingers, and she signed it in her own hand

Valerie Hall

'I hope you can read it,' she said. She was trying to tell me that I had to discover who I am, then the rest *had* to follow, as night must day, if only I could choose to be who I found myself to be. And because of what Val and I had done together, anything could be done. Possibility. That light at the end of the tunnel wasn't just another train coming to mow me down.

'Paul, what you've done for me is you've helped me find my way through,' she said, and turned further away. We were separating. 'And now here I am, almost at the other end.' She sat there for a while, disease-ridden, and leaning back on sterile pillows.

She then turned to me and said, 'I believe I can make my own way from here.' She gave that little nod.

I nodded back, 'Yes, you can. I can see that, Val.' And with that I had accepted. She had given me this one final chance to love her, and without knowing that this was what I was facing, I found I could do it. In the end. Finally.

'And I want you to know,' she said, voice shaking, grey hands flat on sheeted lap, 'that when you die, I'm going to be waiting for you.' She paused for breath and strength. 'And if they'll let me, I'm going to guide you through on the other side.' That's when the tears came.

If you had been watching from the bed next door, you would have seen the old woman raise her arms towards the young man, who leaned forward to hold her. You might have noticed too that they patted each other on the back very gently, very appreciatively, in perfect syncopation. You might even have heard them say that final word, 'Goodbye', in a tearful unison. You would have seen the young man pick up a large well-read book from her bed, and walk out of the ward without looking back. And you would have heard his shoes squeak down the corridors, and away, as *the silence surged softly backward*. If you then had turned to look at that old woman, what would you have seen?

'Val is dead,' I thought. It was the morning of Val and Tom's 53rd wedding anniversary, April Fool's Day. The hospice rang to tell me Val had 'died quietly in her sleep during the night'. I wondered whether they would have told me if she had died screaming and thrashing and yelling abuse.

'She has just died', I thought, trying to make it real. I repeated the same thing to myself, over and over, until I realised that somewhere within I had already known.

'. . . in her sleep'. Had she crossed the bridge during the night? Had she stood over the Silent Pond one final time, and gone on to discover? Or charged the great white horse over the precipice? Or had Val merely faded into oblivion for eternity, another meaningless existence dispassionately extinguished?

And who would notice? There was now a bed temporarily empty in a hospice, a house temporarily unoccupied in her town. But these were the only definite effects her death would have. These were the only ways in which Val could have been seen to be in the way of anybody else.

I sat and searched inwardly for the gap I had been taught must appear, now Val was dead. And I found not that but a full pressure of gratitude in my chest. I sat in the continuing bond with Val, full to bursting. I would not move until I had to, so I sat there for maybe fifteen minutes, maybe an hour, I don't know, time didn't matter. My beloved Val had done it, she had made it.

And so will we, but I only wonder how?

THE FOLLOWING THURSDAY

Nothing.
Everything.

Adrian Brown was my best friend when I was a little boy. He came from a place called England, but I didn't know why. England was where Coronation Street was. Ena Sharples lived there, and Albert Tatlock, and Minnie Someone. Women wore hairnets and everything was in black and white. Adrian Brown talked funny, and so did his mum and dad. Adrian Brown called them 'mummy' and 'daddy', which I thought was stupid. Adrian Brown and I used to play together a lot, but his 'mummy' would never let me have a pee in their toilet – she called it 'The Loo'. So I would have to walk home to Hawera Road to pee, and then go back to Adrian Brown's house to keep playing. In England you couldn't use other people's toilets, only your own. I didn't know why. Then one day they told me Adrian Brown was going back to England to live and Adrian Brown and I were really sad. Then one day Adrian Brown didn't come to school. He wasn't in the line outside our classroom, and he didn't come late either. And when I walked past his house on the way home, I could feel the house was empty. Then on another day I walked past Adrian Brown's house and other people were living there, and so I didn't like them and I tried not to look at the house when I walked to school or when I walked home. But sometimes I looked, and it was an awful feeling, as if there was some sort of worrying hole where Adrian Brown should have been. I didn't know where Adrian Brown was anymore.

This Thursday, I wouldn't be going to Val's house. But there wasn't a hole, there was a beginning.

Part Four

Amen

LEGIONNAIRE
1987

I lay flat out and sweating, a captor of the predatory hospital bed. My temperature was one degree away from leaving me permanently brain-damaged. My then wife and my mother had been told I would probably die that night. Unless you change your direction, a Chinese saying goes, you are likely to end up where you are headed. I was not aware of my mortal predicament; I hadn't been told. As far as I knew I was just extremely exhausted, and my life would go on swimmingly, after I'd had enough rest.

By my late twenties I was, according to colleagues and friends, very successful. Yet I was not as good as most at convincing myself I was happy. An achiever, an exemplary citizen, things had been going well for me, in a societal sense. People generally insisted this was so, but on the night I was to die of Legionnaires' Disease everyone was keeping quiet.

It was ten years after I had nearly drowned, and by this time I had completely lost my reference points. There was no space in my philosophies for death. Death was, after all, unproductive. Or so I thought.

I was restoring a turn of the century villa. The dust was so atrocious I had often left the house to wheeze and gag, eventually developing a cough that wouldn't be shaken off. After much prodding from those around me, I finally conceded that a visit to the doctor wouldn't be amiss. I was examined, I was rushed to x-ray, I was rushed to hospital in an ambulance, and none of these things were what I had thought would happen next in my life.

Being trollied and bumped around the corridors of the hospital was quite exciting. I felt relieved, found. I had been trying too hard, and suddenly it felt as if I'd been rescued from seas too dark and vast, plucked from the malevolent swell by a benevolent hand. I was being given respite, a chance for peace.

They monitored me constantly, invasively, such a nuisance when I was so exhausted. I just wanted to rest, to sleep, forever. I'd had more than enough. That was when my wife and my mother were told I might not make it through the night. I was slowly drowning, the inside of my lungs covered in phlegm. No rocks to cling to.

To the side of my metal hospital bed they came, frightened. They stood there, they tried their best. The smiles on their faces juxtaposed with the fear in their eyes. I couldn't figure them out, and I was dead beat, so I asked them to leave. They said goodbye and told me they would visit the following day, but they weren't sure that was going to happen. No one pointed this out. They thought that would be best. Maybe they were right. Maybe not knowing helped save me.

The doctors did not tell me I was dying, nor the nurses, nor anyone else who was caring for me. My temperature soaring, I felt frozen to the marrow and shook violently from head to toe. Utterly exposed and vulnerable, I fell in love that night with the nurse who tended me as I lay there, dying. She tenderly wiped away my sweat; she patiently raised me up to drink; she uncomplainingly changed my sheets in the middle of the night; she gently changed my drip; but of all the blessings she bestowed it was the touching of my skin and the stroking of my hair that helped me feel human. The little equilibrium I'd had within myself was gone; it was Her I clung to now. I reached out; I held on; I gasped for air.

I awoke the next morning. My temperature had lowered, and the doctors seemed as bewildered as I had been throughout the night. I had clearly rallied, but they were having difficulty discovering exactly how they had brought this about. It didn't occur to them that it could have been the night nurse, holding my hand.

I lay still in bed, turned towards the adjoining hall, longing for her to come back to me in the ward. I lay silently, waiting. Everyone else was a disappointment. I waited days and nights, telling no one, and she did not come. It was only a one-night stand, but I believe she saved me.

I was still dazed and confused when, after a few days, I was told I could leave the hospital. A doctor glanced through my medical notes and pronounced I'd suffered a bad chest infection, was f.i.n.e. (Fucked up, Insecure, Neurotic, and Emotional) now, and should be gone. He snapped my file shut.

'My GP told me I'd had Legionnaires' Disease,' I said hesitantly, staring at the cardboard file.

'Oh,' he said, fumbling internally and externally, and

bravely reopened my file. He rapidly regained his posturing gravity and certainty, as if he were a judge at my trial. He turned to another page in the file, not the one I'd been reading upside down. 'Ah yes . . .' he opened brilliantly to the defendant. It was as if he had at last discovered the truth, through a remarkable piece of deduction that had been significantly hampered in the first place by my impertinent questions.

'Yes, you've had Legionnaires' Disease. But you're alright now. And at least you can rest assured you will never get it again.' He pronounced his judgement confidently, beaming down into the accused.

'If everyone who has had this disease before has died,' I said to him as I thought aloud, 'then how can you know it isn't possible for me to catch it again?' He seemed surprised and annoyed that I could think, and closed his file. 'Rest assured!' he said, but he didn't say about what. He rose from his chair and showed me out.

I rested restlessly for weeks in the house that had almost killed me, contemplating the lifeless life I was cured to return to, awaiting the return each evening of a partner I could barely communicate with. It wasn't her fault; it was ours. My 'life', and I use the word in its loosest possible sense, went on in the same vein for another year. I returned to work after a three-month convalescence, doing a well-paid job and wondering why. Then one day my boss, Terry, called me into his office to tell me that now he was sixty-two years of age, he wanted to retire and have me take over the business. He sat there and offered me three times my salary, a new car (every year), round the world travel (every year), an open-

ended expense account at the local liquor store (every day –
I'd need it), his office, his problems, his life (he didn't mention
the last two).

When he had finished laying it all out, he leaned back in
his big creaking leather chair. He folded his hands confidently
over his large stomach, raised his eyebrows, and smiled warmly
down into me, as I sat on the little chair on the other side of
the broad shiny desk. *My* desk. I was twenty-nine years old.
Everything I had worked towards was being offered to me
on a plate.

I resigned on the spot.

Terry was shocked. So was everyone else I left. I resigned
from that whole life, on the spot. I had finally, hopefully,
realised in that moment that I was trapped in a continuing
despair. I left my job of seven years, my career, and someone
else's future. I left my wife, my fashionable villa, my friends.
I abandoned that life, and with it forfeited its secure depend-
able future: the dinners with people I would pretend knew
me; buying new sofas and bedspreads and redecorating the
house; following the local sports team; developing my palate
for wine; using the jogging machine at the gym. I gathered
about a thousand dollars, I bought a one-way ticket to the
other side of the world, and I used it.

I arrived in London at the end of April 1988, two weeks
before my thirtieth birthday. The day was grey and cold and
nothing was anything like I was used to. My brother John and
his wife Maree met me at Heathrow airport and drove me
through the most depressing rows of houses I'd ever seen. It
wasn't their size or design that got to me, it was the uniformity,

the implicit conformity. Row after row of the same, repli-
cated for millions. My heart sank into my stomach as we
drove, hemmed in by these dehumanising buildings. I felt a
pull towards all I had left behind. What had I *done*?

I got an urgent phone call from New Zealand. Terry was
ill and couldn't work anymore – would I come back and take
the job he had offered me. A second chance. I did not go
back. And Terry died.

A chasm opened up before me as I was faced with the
result of disposing of the life I had had: the utter humanity
of facing the unknown. It is with respect and a huge amount
of gratitude, that I can now look back at that younger Paul.
With nothing to cling to, he relinquished all that he could.
He went over the precipice, not with a reining in but at a
gallop, to leap and fall into the hands of the Gods.

DEAD CHUFFED
April 1995

I arrived for Val's funeral early, and hung around outside the crematorium like a lost soul before going in. I was surprised at the number of people. There were thirty or so, including nurses from the hospice and volunteers from the charity. Some of these people had only heard stories about Val during their training with me. I wondered if Christine had heard of her mother's death, if she was there; I wondered, but it didn't seem to matter.

Val had wanted to be cremated, not buried. The pond was the last hole that would be dug for her, 'with the small end pointing towards the house'. Pop would have dug a small hole for her in his back yard. Dad dug holes too. The house on Hawera Road was all on one level, and the family was rapidly expanding. To make room for more kids, dad dug underneath the house. First he made a cellar, then like Pop, he dug bigger holes. First a garage, big enough for two cars, then a hole big enough for a bedroom for me and John.

Pop dug holes, and dad dug holes, so we kids began to dig holes. John and I and the boys from next door, we dug a tunnel in the cellar. When dad found it he was really angry. We had dug our tunnel under the foundations of the house.

And there was this paving stone that mum stood on to hang the washing out in the back garden. We pulled up the stone slab and dug a hole under it. We got a little box and put things in it that would not be found for a hundred years, when everyone would be living on the moon and wear little televisions on their wrists. In the box we put the front page of the *New Zealand Herald*, a toy gun (broken), a Vegemite sandwich, and stuff like that. We laid the stone back down, trying not to crunch the bugs that had come out of nowhere to swarm around the hole. We got a real telling off about that hole too. It was Dangerous.

Pop dug holes, dad dug holes, and I dug the hole for Val's pond. But there was to be no hole for Val.

I sat there in the chapel, thinking of holes and waiting. I didn't feel like a mourner as such, but a celebrant. I was not sad or grief-stricken that Val had died, I was grateful that I had known her, and that I'd known her at a most significant time in her life.

On entering, I didn't cross myself, but my body could not help itself stooping a little in the direction of the altar – operant conditioning, Pavlov's dog. I looked around the gathering for familiar faces, and chose to sit on my own.

There were the usual punitive wooden benches, and on sitting down I saw Val looking back from the altar rail. She was perched irreverently, legs swinging back and forth as she faced the crowd she had drawn, *her* crowd. The late Val Hall had the ageless quality she had developed of late, but even more so, being every age between a child and an elderly woman. This had struck me about her from the time she had said to me, 'I'm Me! I'm just me. And I love it.' The late Val Hall.

There she was, on the brink, right in front of everyone, where only I could see her. She looked dead chuffed with herself. The vicar turned up on stage and began speaking in a clear voice with an expression of solemn confidence – he had never met Val. Val shrugged and, with a raise of her eyebrow, was gone.

The service went on until a respectful enough amount of time had been used up, then we filed outside, heads down, trying not to look too pleased with ourselves for turning up. I was accosted by people wanting to know if I was Paul, 'Val has said so much about you'. I nodded politely, perhaps ungraciously, and retreated to my old car.

I drove to Val's house for the last time. The anonymous nondescript little house where there had been so much space and time within the meagre time and space we'd had. I stood amongst the throng of people in a tiny lifeless room that looked out to a rectangular garden on the verge of a missed spring.

I kept looking over to the sofa, and was about to leave when someone said to me, 'Paul, have you met Christine?'

And there she was, a diminutive woman, a young dark-haired Val. I could immediately see in her eyes and the set of her chin that she had no regrets and would make no apologies or excuses. When asked to summarise his existential classic *L'Etranger*, Albert Camus said, 'In our society any man who doesn't cry at his mother's funeral is liable to be condemned to death.' Christine was definitely up for it.

'Hello,' she said, shaking my hand a little too firmly. 'People have been telling me about you.'

'I'm glad you were able to come,' I said, 'Will you be staying here?'

'I'm in a hotel not too far.' Enough said. I was surprised that I felt no animosity towards her, but a strange sort of sympathy. Val had not been much of a mother to this person, I knew that, and nothing had been magically wiped out or resolved through Val's death. I didn't see Christine in the chapel, but if she did not cry I for one would not condemn her for it.

'What will you do with the house?' I said, the home where she had been raised, the root of her childhood.

'It's already on the market.' Very matter-of-fact, very Val. In her defiant position Christine had become, as is always the case in such protests, even more defined by Val. It seemed to me that it was Val, not Christine herself, who had remained Christine's reference point, despite her attempts to reorient herself.

'There are a couple of things I want for myself,' she said, 'but there's nothing else.' I had the impression that this was a woman who had done a great deal of talking to someone about her upbringing.

'It was good to have the chance to meet you, Christine,' I said. 'I'll be off now. Goodbye and good luck to you.'

She caught my eyes and I saw her ambivalence in that moment, as if she wanted something but feared what the gaining of it might mean. So I paused. I wasn't aware Christine had a note from Val, a note suggesting Christine speak to me about the end of Val's life. Nevertheless, I had decided that if Christine were to ask me, I would tell her all about it, otherwise I would hold my tongue. I'd become rather adept at this. I waited for that full long-setting second as I held her eye.

'Goodbye,' she said, and I left that empty house, finally.

I sat outside in the car, as I'd always done after a visit, following the rituals to the last, completing the circle. I remembered Val's face poking through the net curtains as I crossed the road with the shopping trolley, wobbly-weighted with soaking sand. I started up my old VW and drove off down the quiet road. It was lined with its little nondescript houses, occupied by people seemingly unruffled by the fact that they were heading irretrievably towards their deaths.

POSTMORTEM

1995

Tom, Val's husband, had liked motorcycles – Enfields. I liked Harleys. I'd liked them from the first time I saw *Easy Rider*; I liked the bike with the flames on the tank. Like the flames on my surfboard. I bought my first motorcycle when I was fifteen. It was a little Suzuki 125, and I had worked for years in a Chinese fruit and vegetable shop to save the money. Malo Jay means Monkey Boy. That's what they called me in the shop, Malo Jay. Dad said he would put in as much money as I saved, even though he didn't like motorcycles. Dad could be good like that.

Even if I saw one cent on the footpath, I'd bend down to pick it up. It didn't matter who I was with, it was a gift and I'd take it. Eventually I had enough money, and I bought that little red Suzuki and taught myself to ride.

Dad liked that I worked hard and saved my money to buy Things. I would see him looking at his new golf clubs, or his new stereo, or his new car, and the way he looked at them I knew he would never look at me that way. So I turned to Things as well. I had this little red Suzuki 125 I had saved for for years, and John got on it and rode it straight through the hedge and scratched it. I was gutted.

Things were beginning to mean everything to me.

Then I saved some more money, and I bought a bigger bike. Dad didn't like it. He said my motorcycle friends were 'Yahoos'. My sister Mary had never ridden on a motorcycle before, so one day I took her out on mine. We rode straight into the side of a VW Beetle. As we hit the car I was only a few feet from the driver, who was looking straight ahead as he drove merrily through the Give Way intersection without looking. I went over the roof of the Beetle, and landed on the road and was knocked out. Mary went over the roof of the Beetle and landed on me and bounced off. The skin on her fingers was scraped off on the hard surface of the road, like mine had been underwater, clinging to the rocks. The motorbike, a big Suzuki 400 trail bike, went over the roof of the Beetle and landed on me as well. I was told this when I woke up on the road. When I was taken away in the ambulance I was really worried about my bike. Things had come to mean almost everything to me.

So it was a while before I rode my Harley to Val's. Motorcycle riders are Yahoos. I didn't know what she would think of her hospice visitor turning up on a motorbike. 'You'll have to take me for a ride,' she said.

I hadn't been expecting that. But that's how I found out Tom liked Enfields. And that's how I found out it might not matter so much what I appeared to be, it was more important who I was. And being with Val, I thought I was getting to grips with loss. Until one day I lost one of my motorcycle gloves in a book store. This glove meant much more to me than I thought. It was like a companion, somehow. And what use was one without the other. And when I felt how much it hurt to lose it, then I knew a little more about loss. Val and I, in the end, we fitted together like hand in glove. Then one was lost.

In a warm and sympathetic letter of condolence to the widow of Binswanger, Sigmund Freud wrote:

Although we know that after such a loss the acute state of mourning will subside, we also know we shall remain inconsolable and will never find a substitute. No matter what may fill the gap, even if it be filled completely, it nevertheless remains something else. And actually this is how it should be. It is the only way of perpetuating that love which we do not want to relinquish.

I don't agree with Freud on this and many other issues, as it seems to me to be a requirement, an injunction of our culture, that 'we shall remain inconsolable' when someone we love dies. That we 'will never find a substitute' may be true, but why should we? Were they not enough? And the proposition that 'the only way of perpetuating that love' is not to fill the gap is, to my mind, against Nature. Val was dead and I was not inconsolable, even though I had finally, fleetingly, truly and unreservedly loved her. And the ending of her life filled a gap, rather than left one. My love for Val lives on, in and of itself, and, I hope, through my psychotherapy patients and students.

By May, spring had sprung, the air awash with neophytic life. The doorbell rang. 'Delivery for a Mister McDermott'. I trekked down the three flights of stairs, to be handed a box of plants.

'Um, are you sure these are for me?' I said. A puzzle.

'This you, is it?' the man said, showing me my name on the delivery slip. Yes, it was. 'You might have forgot ordering them, mate,' he said as he shuffled some papers. 'Right, it says here they were ordered in February.'

A hot full flush of recognition spread from my neck to my cheeks. 'Ah!' I said in perfect French, 'Thanks, mate'. I took the cardboard box of new life up and out to the roof terrace, and put them gently down on the sun-warmed wooden decking. I sat down beside them, with them, and stared up at the sky for a while. Val. I'd never liked geraniums, but that didn't matter; Val thought I liked them because she did.

And that was, in one sense, the end. But it wasn't a full stop, only a comma. As it was in the beginning, is now and ever shall be: World without end. We were fortunate, Val and I, that we had not begun with certainties, for that would only have ended in doubts. We were content to begin with doubts, with puzzles. So in the end, when we knew, then we knew that we knew. As Herman Hesse wrote in *Journey To The East*:

> *We had within us something stronger than reality or probability, and that was faith in the meaning and necessity of our action.*

I wish you could have met Val, you'd have liked her,

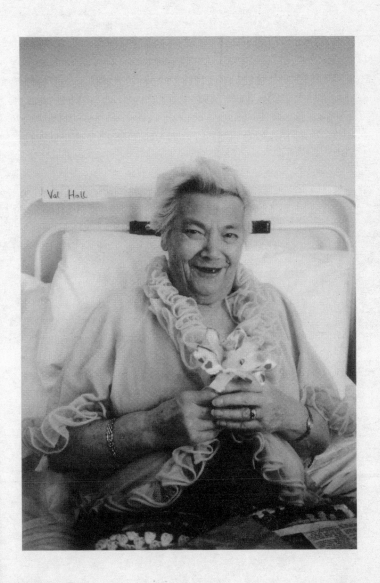

Val Hall

ACKNOWLEDGEMENTS

In writing this book I walked up to a wall, with the intention of walking through it. I didn't think I could do it, but I understood that I would. And on the way I had some help. I want to thank Anthony Lunt for his insights into my relationship with Val, in particular my last meeting with her, and for bringing my feet nearer to the ground, my heart closer to others, and my eyes towards the Heavens. I thank Debbie Charles for telling me her dream, as it brought within it all the permission I needed. And I am grateful to Cary McDermott and Ali Glenny for their encouragement and fruitful criticism.

When you're inside the wall it is very dark, and it can be lonely. You have to have faith to keep going. And you need to harness your intent when opportunities appear and the moments are ripe, or else you won't get through. And there was Anthony again, constant; and Judith Kendra of Rider Books with her thoughtful and encouraging surgery; and Pili Perez-Roel and Rebecca Miskin when and where I most needed them, with a pat on the back, a soft kind word and lashings of Rioja.

And when you're coming out the other side of the wall, you have to check you're still all there; that you haven't lost anything important or, worse still, gained anything that isn't. Thanks also to those who will be there on that side of the wall, when this end becomes a beginning. And that, I believe, may be the most difficult thing of all.